T0280632

Ruptured Uterus

Gowri Dorairajan

Ruptured Uterus

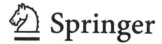 Springer

Gowri Dorairajan
Obstetrics and Gynecology
JIPMER
Puducherry
India

ISBN 978-981-10-9720-1   ISBN 978-981-10-2852-6   (eBook)
DOI 10.1007/978-981-10-2852-6

Printed on acid-free paper

This Springer imprint is published by Springer Nature
The registered company is Springer Science+Business Media Singapore Pte Ltd.
The registered company address is 152 Beach Road, #22-06/08 Gateway East, Singapore 189721, Singapore

I dedicate this book to those agonized labouring women who could never take their babies back home with them, to the family of the labouring women who never went back home after delivery, and to those who would never experience a baby growing within them again. I dedicate this to those who forgave and healed and to those who could not forget and carried the scar.

I dedicate this to all obstetricians who had experienced the triumph when the baby cried happily, when the mother was thankful, and when they averted what could otherwise have been a very bad obstetric nightmare: all this when the world slept peacefully. I dedicate this to all those who thought they did their best possible at that time but realized late that they could have done better.

I dedicate this book to all my teachers and seniors only the goodness of whom I have nurtured as glowing lamps within me. I dedicate this book to all those caregivers who lost their health during their journey. I dedicate this to those yearning students who wanted readable understandable and effective methods of learning and those who wished the experience of grey hair would translate into black and white print.

I dedicate this book to the divine power whose presence I have experienced while managing labouring women. I pray that the students of obstetrics would become competent, compassionate, caring, and careful obstetricians. Each one of us should become comrades to the juniors and pass on the baton wholeheartedly and selflessly to win the relay race of obstetrics.

I pray to God that every individual would wholesomely heal.

With attitude of gratitude,

Gowri Dorairajan

Preface

One learns from teachers to graduate, from books during post-graduation, and from patients to become an experienced specialist.

Most of the textbooks have a chapter on ruptured uterus where the classical symptoms and signs are enumerated. I have worked in various hospitals in various capacities. While working, I came across many cases of ruptured uterus. Each case had something different. In many of these cases, the classical symptoms and signs were hidden, and various features camouflaged the classical ones. These different features act as a background for the chameleon of ruptured uterus to change its colour, and spotting the chameleon or in other words diagnosing the rupture becomes a challenge.

I conceived this book to bridge the experience gap among those who work day in and out in the emergency rooms and labour rooms. I have therefore narrated the cases I came across over the last 25 years to bring out the different colours of presentation of ruptured uterus. The details presented would help the practitioners of obstetrics to relate to the cases and become aware of the various manifestations of ruptured uterus and hence have a high index of suspicion for ruptured uterus. For this reason, some of the photographs have been photoshopped to depict the scenarios that happened many years back because the intraoperative documentation was not easy those days and most of them are vividly imprinted only in my memory.

The literature on ruptured uterus is extensive. There are many guidelines available for selecting and monitoring cases for TOLAC. I have brought these wherever appropriate. I have also quoted many cases from literature to complete the possible aetiologies, presentations, and management of ruptured uterus.

Puducherry, India   Gowri Dorairajan

Acknowledgements

I would like to thank my patients for allowing me to be a part of their journey in life. I would like to thank my students for inspiring me to narrate my experience in the form of a book.

I would like to thank my teachers who have inspired me during my journey. I thank my family for adjusting with me for snatching away their time that should have been spent with me as I wrote the book.

I thank Almighty for helping me conceive this book at this juncture of my journey and all the help that came my way to complete it.

I thank my colleagues for sharing a few of the intraoperative photographs.

I thank my computer technicians for patiently helping me.

Contents

About the Author

The author Dr. Gowri Dorairajan is a professor and head of a unit at JIPMER, Puducherry, which is an autonomous institute of national importance. Dr. Gowri Dorairajan is an acclaimed teacher and clinician. She has vast experience. She did her post-graduate training from Lady Hardinge Medical College, New Delhi, from 1992 to 1995.

She has gained vast clinical experience by working in various government hospitals with very high turnover of obstetric cases. After completing post MD training for 3 years at the above college, she worked at JIPMER, Puducherry, for 5 years from 1999 to 2004 as a research officer, senior research associate, and then as an assistant professor. Thereafter, she worked as a specialist at Government Maternity Hospital, Puducherry. Working in these three important hospitals with high turnover and over 14000 deliveries a year, she has had vast exposure to various obstetric emergencies and cases.

She joined back JIPMER as professor in the year 2013.

She has over 18 years of teaching experience. She has been a teacher for undergraduate and post-graduate students and DNB trainees. She has guided many students with their thesis and research work over the years. She is well known among the students for her teaching skills.

In the evolving era of technology and imaging, the author feels that the clinical acumen is taking a back seat and feels that it should be strongly imparted and developed in the present-day trainees.

The need to translate the vast clinical experience into black and white knowledge that can be applied into day-to-day action even by the trainee compelled the author to write this book in the present style.

Introduction

1

Ruptured uterus is an obstetric calamity attended with high perinatal mortality and maternal morbidity and mortality.

One usually blames the birth attendants or dais of remote areas for mismanagement as they failed to recognize labour problem and referred the case rather late. In the past, it would typically occur in non-supervised pregnancies and unsupervised labour with the delay in transportation to referral centres. For these reasons, it has been more common in developing countries and not unusual in the emergency obstetric rooms.

However, these time-old factors have been addressed, and the situation has changed. It is a cause for great concern when it happens in the labour wards of tertiary care centres due to the inadvertent and injudicious use of inducing agents and due to unduly prolonged trial of labour in cases with previous caesarean sections. Inappropriate selection of cases of previous caesarean sections for the trial of labour is an important concern in developing countries. The primary caesarean sections are performed in district hospitals or practitioners under various situations leading to an unrealized integrally weak scar getting tested during labour in the subsequent pregnancy.

The list of aetiologies for rupture uterus is however ever increasing. The advances in technologies have only dispelled human endeavour to improve infrastructures and transportation and communication to reduce the rates of neglected labour and artificial reproductive techniques which have opened up a new list of causes of rupture of the uterus, and the list remains exhaustive. At the same time, improved infrastructure and maternal critical care facilities, round-the-clock accessible blood, and its components and antibiotics have reduced the maternal morbidity and mortality over the years.

The chapters that follow narrate the various cases as I came across during the last 20 years of my practice. I have tried to bring out the varied clinical presentations and background settings of the cases. The narration of the cases brings out the need for high index of suspicion for diagnosing ruptured uterus.

© Springer Nature Singapore Pte Ltd. 2017
G. Dorairajan, *Ruptured Uterus*, DOI 10.1007/978-981-10-2852-6_1

The important features are summarized in a point-wise fashion in a box to reinforce the important take-home message from the various clinical situations.

In an interesting study using data from birth registry from Norway, the authors [1] examined the time trends of uterine rupture and observed a sharply increasing rate of rupture from 1.2/10,000 maternities between 1967 and 1977 to 6.1/10,000 maternities from 2000 to 2008. Scarring due to caesarean section, augmentation with oxytocin, and induction with prostaglandins and oxytocin were a few of the factors responsible for the increased rate of rupture. They did observe a decrease in maternal mortality from hysterectomy and postpartum haemorrhage and a decline in intrapartum and infant deaths as a complication of rupture over the decades. Anyone who has been working in obstetric units for more than 10–15 years would agree with this observation.

Reference

1. Al-Zirqi I, Stray-Pedersen B, Forsén L, Daltveit AK, Vangen S. Uterine rupture: trends over 40 years. BJOG. 2015;123(5):780–7. doi:10.1111/1471-0528.13394.

Rupture of the Uterus Scarred Due to Previous Caesarean Section

2

A 24-year-old primigravida married for 1 year was referred from a village in the second stage of labour with an intrauterine foetal demise to the emergency room. There was mild tachycardia. She was not anaemic. The blood pressure was normal. A midline vertical sub-umbilical scar on the abdomen was claimed to be for an ovariotomy done during adolescence. The patient was exhausted. There was secondary inertia of the uterus. Vaginal examination confirmed full dilatation with fully rotated vertex at +2 station. Forceps delivery was uneventfully performed to deliver a 2.8 kg dead baby. Massive postpartum haemorrhage followed the delivery. There was no trauma to the lower genital tract. Since the brisk bleeding very quickly started exsanguinating the patient, she was taken up for urgent laparotomy, only to realize there was transverse rupture of a previous hysterotomy scar (Fig. 2.1).

The rent appeared to be rather high in the lower segment. The rent was repaired. This presentation was the first ever case I saw nearly 23 years back. In this presentation of a ruptured scarred uterus, the foetus was still intrauterine probably because the head and shoulders were deep in the pelvis. The trunk of the foetus must have acted as a tamponade and prevented exsanguination till the uterine contents were emptied vaginally. The women later confirmed hysterotomy for an unwanted pregnancy before wedlock which had been obviously hidden for social reasons.

Previous caesarean scar ruptures are the commonest cause of rupture of the uterus. It can present in various ways.

2.1 Asymptomatic Rupture

The most benign and harmless are those which are recognized as full-thickness rupture at the time of elective repeat caesarean section. Some of these caesarean sections are performed as before labour as emergency caesarean section due to suprapubic pain or unexplained tachycardia. Qureshi [35] had graded the intraoperative scars into four grades. Grades III and IV (incomplete or complete

© Springer Nature Singapore Pte Ltd. 2017
G. Dorairajan, *Ruptured Uterus*, DOI 10.1007/978-981-10-2852-6_2

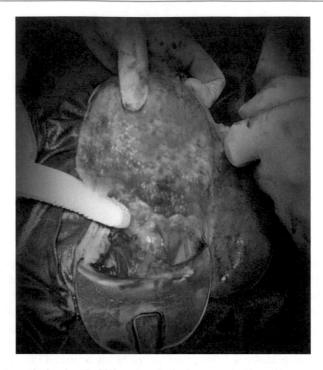

Fig. 2.1 Photograph showing the high rupture in the lower segment

dehiscence) are occasionally observed in elective caesarean sections. Fortunately, the maternal as well as foetal outcome is unaffected in such situations.

With the rising caesarean section rate in the last two decades, one is likely to encounter pregnancies with previous caesarean sections. Scar rupture among women undergoing labour after previous caesarean sections has varied presentations.

Women with previous caesarean during labour should be carefully and diligently monitored. The decision for allowing them to labour either spontaneous or induced should be taken with prudence.

2.2   Scar Rupture During Labour

2.2.1   Scar Rupture in the First Stage of Labour

A woman was being supervised in her second pregnancy in our antenatal clinic. In her first pregnancy two and a half years back, a caesarean section had been performed for foetal distress during labour at term at a private nursing home. The baby had weighed 2.8 kg and was doing well. The caesarean operation and the postoperative recovery were uneventful. In the present pregnancy, there were no comorbidities or any complications. The foetus was in left occipito-anterior position, and the

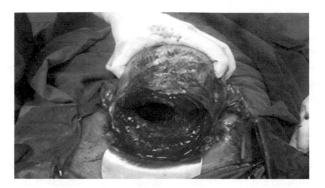

Fig. 2.2 Intraoperative photograph showing full-thickness scar rupture after delivering the foetus

estimated birth weight was 2.7 kg. The pelvis was normal. She was willing for the trial of labour (TOLAC), and so we waited for spontaneous labour. The woman came back in spontaneous labour and was admitted in active labour. At admission, her pulse rate was 84/min with normal blood pressure. Abdomen revealed single-term foetus in left occipito-anterior position with regular good uterine contractions. The foetal heart trace was good. Vaginal examination confirmed 4 cm dilatation with full effacement and clear liquor draining. The pelvis was adequate, and the vertex was at -2 station. Two hours later she suddenly developed tachycardia with foetal bradycardia. The cervix was 6 cm and vertex was at -1 station, but the liquor was meconium stained. She was taken up for immediate caesarean section; there was full-thickness full-length scar rupture (Fig. 2.2). We delivered an asphyxiated 2.8 kg foetus from within the uterus. The rent was repaired.

The baby died in the NICU after 24 h. I felt miserable about the decision. Later I got to know that in that nursing home as a matter of routine, caesareans were performed by surgeons who would close uterus in single-layer locking sutures. Over a period, we have learnt lessons by facing the mishaps of rupture and scar dehiscence. We have identified the hospitals and the nursing homes surrounding our hospital whose caesarean scars have failed to withstand labour. We no longer post the women who underwent caesareans in these hospitals for TOLAC. It is a cause of great concern as there is an increase in the rate of repeat caesareans for fear of rupture. It is the moral and ethical duty of those who perform primary caesareans to follow the scientific techniques of repairing the incision and documenting the same properly in the discharge slips.

The commonest reason for concern suspecting the integrity of the scar is maternal tachycardia. However, there may be situations when one may take the decision to deliver by caesarean due to maternal tachycardia only to find a healthy intact previous scar. It is, therefore, important to give adequate pain relief and keep her well hydrated to prevent tachycardia due to other reasons confusing the picture.

Pain in the suprapubic region is another symptom of concern and might be one of the reasons for performing an emergency caesarean section. Cohen and colleagues [13] observed that abdominal pain alone is a poor predictor of scar rupture, but in the presence of an additional symptom or sign, it has a nearly 60% positive predictive value for rupture.

It is also commonplace to find foetal heart rate abnormalities as the most important and only manifestation of scar dehiscence. Quite often during monitoring, one finds foetal tachycardia, variable deceleration, or bradycardia in a labouring woman with a previous caesarean scar.

In a population-based case-control study among women with previous caesarean section undergoing a trial of labour, Andersen and co-authors [5] observed that 77. 5% of women with rupture had pathological (cardiotocography) CTG in early labour. Foetal tachycardia was significantly higher in women with scar rupture than in controls (OR=2.5). Severe recurrent variable decelerations were also found to predict rupture.

In a large multicenter case-control study [16], the authors observed that grade 3 foetal heart abnormalities (as defined by the FIGO guidelines [17]), in a woman with a previous caesarean scar in labour, are significantly likely to be associated with scar dehiscence, with an odds ratio of 4.1. It is important to view the foetal heart rate abnormality seriously and consider termination by caesarean section instead of an overenthusiastic attempt at resuscitation and continuing the trial because though the foetal heart rate may transiently recover, it may present a little later as a florid rupture where the risk of losing the baby increases many times. In this regard, the American [1] Royal College of Obstetrics and Gynaecology [36] and the Canadian Society [44] have recommended the use of continuous electronic foetal heart rate monitoring in women undergoing a trial of labour after previous caesarean section.

The other manifestation of scar dehiscence during labour is bleeding from the vagina. Typically it may not be excessive. Sometimes it may be perceived as the excessive show. Patients with abruption may further confuse the picture. That brings me to this case. A woman presented at 34 weeks of pregnancy with acute onset bleeding. It was the first episode associated with diffuse abdominal pain. There was a loss of foetal movements. She was in her second pregnancy and had one live issue. Previous was a caesarean section done in a private hospital for foetal distress. On examination she was pale. The pulse rate was 110/min. The blood pressure was 100/60 mm of Hg. The abdomen revealed a 36-week size uterus that was tense and tender. The foetal heart sound was absent. The uterine contour was made out, and the uterus was contracting. There was haematuria. Scar rupture was a close differential diagnosis, but because of the uterus acting and relaxing, it was less likely. On pelvic examination the cervix was 2 cm; 50% effaced, membranes were present with the vertex at -3 station. Artificial rupture of membranes confirmed blood-stained liquor. Thus, the working diagnosis was grade IIIb abruption. The labour was augmented with low-dose oxytocin, and parallel resuscitation and correction of coagulation failure were carried out. Thus, it is very important to understand that even though there may be maternal tachycardia, bleeding, foetal demise, and haematuria in a woman with previous caesarean section, other causes like abruption could be an underlying feature, and the fact that uterus is contracting and relaxing may be the only feature against scar dehiscence.

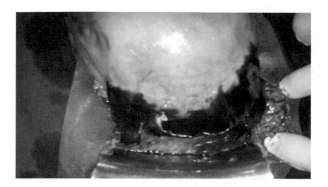

Fig. 2.3   Photograph showing bruising of the entire lower segment

She eventually delivered, but there was a continuous trickle of bleed with the uterus having a tendency to relax. The scar appeared thinned at digital exploration. Given continued postpartum haemorrhage and suspected scar integrity, she was taken up for laparotomy. Strangely the whole lower segment was bruised (Fig. 2.3).

There was couvelaire uterus. The utero-vesical fold was opened. The bruised lower segment was freshened and sutured. She recovered well. Whether the bruising was a manifestation of coagulation failure or impending rupture is a debatable issue.

A woman presented in labour at term. Her previous delivery was by lower segment caesarean section 3 years back for non-progress of labour in a government hospital. It was a 3 kg baby. The postoperative period was uneventful. At the time of admission, the pulse rate was 84/min. There was a single foetus in right occipito-anterior position palpable three-fifths above the brim. The expected foetal weight was 2.7 kg. The contractions were regular and moderate. Vaginal examination revealed 4 cm dilated fully effaced well-applied cervix. The clear amniotic fluid was draining, and membranes were absent. The position was confirmed as ROA and the station was -2. The pelvis was normal. She was monitored closely for the progress of labour. The foetal heart rate was well preserved with good variability and no decelerations. Two hours later the contractions seemed to become less intense and regular. The frequency reduced to once in 4 min and would last only 25 s. There was no maternal tachycardia. Foetal heart trace was good. Vaginal examination revealed a protracted dilation and descent. Labour was augmented with low-dose oxytocin drip. The contractions transiently improved in intensity but became erratic with few contractions lacking the intensity and remaining ill-sustained. Labour augmentation was continued while the woman and the foetus were carefully monitored. The foetal heart trace was well preserved; there was no maternal tachycardia or bleeding from the vagina. After 2 h vaginal examination revealed arrested dilation and descent, and so the decision for termination by caesarean section was taken. There was scar rupture of 1 cm length at the right end with the loss of all the layers and the foetal head seen through (Fig. 2.4). The foetus was delivered in good condition, and the rent was repaired. The recovery was uneventful.

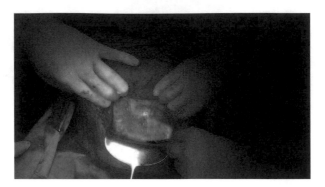

Fig. 2.4 Intraoperative photograph showing the full-thickness scar dehiscence

I wonder if there was any further prolongation, there might have been a full-blown rupture affecting the foetal outcome. It is extremely important to be vigilant about the changing patterns of uterine contractions in a woman with previous caesarean scars. In the above case, there was no maternal tachycardia or bleeding or foetal heart rate abnormities. Any incoordinate uterine contractions or tendency for secondary inertia might be the only subtle sign of early dehiscence as in this case.

Thus, diligent monitoring of various possible manifestations (Box 2.1) of a scar giving way is very important during the first stage of labour.

Box 2.1 Features of Scar Dehiscence in the First Stage of Labour
Maternal tachycardia
Suprapubic pain
Vaginal bleeding
Foetal heart rate abnormalities
Incoordinate uterine contractions
Secondary uterine inertia
Haematuria

2.2.2   Scar Rupture in the Second Stage of Labour

The second stage is a particularly testing period for the strength of the scar. For this reason, some authors [22] have advocated forceps delivery to cut short the second stage of labour.

I have come across many cases where caesarean was decided for the non-descent of the head with deceleration even in the second stage to realize that there was scar dehiscence at the time of caesarean delivery.

This particular case I now narrate is just to discourage heroic decisions. A 28-year-old second gravida was supervised from the early pregnancy. She had undergone a caesarean 3 years back in our hospital for foetal distress to deliver a

3 kg baby. The records confirmed an uneventful lower segment caesarean section, and the incision had been closed in two layers. The postpartum recovery was uneventful. In the ongoing pregnancy, there were no comorbidities. She crossed her dates and would not go into labour. It was a 3.5 kg expected birth weight. The pelvis was normal and adequate. The foetus was in occipito-transverse position at -3 station. In an attempt to reduce the caesarean section rate, it was decided to induce labour as everything was conducive and the woman was willing for TOLAC. The cervix was ripened with Foleys catheter bulb. Labour was induced with a low dose of oxytocin. Active labour got established though it became slightly protracted. Labour augmentation was continued with oxytocin in spite of the protracted labour. The foetal heart was well preserved, and the liquor was clear. She achieved the second stage. There was an arrest of descent of the head beyond +1 station even after 1 h of being in the second stage. Foetal bradycardia was noticed, and she was taken up for caesarean section. There was a full-thickness scar rupture. A 3.75 kg stillborn foetus was extracted, and the uterus was repaired. It is prudent to consider elective caesarean section if the baby weight is on the higher side. As I already brought out, the other important though subtle signals we need to be watchful about are protracted labour, after she has achieved active labour especially so with a baby weight on the higher side. In a nested case-control study by Harper et al. [23], the authors observed that women who had scar rupture or failed TOLAC had protracted progress after 7 cm dilation.

2.2.3   Scar Rupture Diagnosed Postpartum

Scar rupture at the second stage may have varied presentations. I came across an extremely interesting case. A woman with previous caesarean section presented to the hospital in labour. She was found to have severe preeclampsia. The previous caesarean was done 2 years back for a nonrecurring indication. At the time of admission, she was not pale. The blood pressure was 160/ 100 mm of Hg. She was 4 cm dilated with good foetal heart sounds and a 2.5 kg expected baby weight. Artificial rupture of membranes revealed clear liquor. The labour progressed well, and she delivered a 2.6 kg baby uneventfully spontaneously after 4 h of admission. There was no postpartum haemorrhage. The blood pressure settled.

After 12–14 h of delivery, she developed mild abdominal distension and pain. The pulse rate was 100 per minute. She did not appear pale. The blood pressure was 130/80 mm of Hg. The abdomen was mildly distended and tender but not guarded. Urine was mildly high coloured, and output was around 40 ml per hour. We observed the patient and infused fluids. Sonography revealed slight free fluid in the abdomen, but all other organs were normal. There was no bowel dilatation observed. The uterus was puerperal with an empty cavity. The abdominal girth slowly increased, and she developed tachypnoea. Abdominal paracentesis revealed haemoperitoneum. At laparotomy, there was a complete full-length scar rupture. The edges had retracted, and there was slow ooze from the edges. The presentation could be as indolent as this with a good perinatal outcome.

In yet another case, I was called by the registrar from the family planning operation theatre. She was doing puerperal sterilization for a woman who had a successful, uneventful vaginal birth after caesarean section (VBAC) 2 days ago with us in the hospital. The registrar suspected something wrong because haemoperitoneum showed up even on opening the abdomen by mini-laparotomy incision. On extending the abdominal incision, a full-length complete rupture became evident; the margins had nearly stopped oozing on their own. The same was easily repaired. How lucky are a few patients and how varied is the presentation of scar rupture that follows delivery of the foetus!

As illustrated by the above two cases, the scar can rupture late in the second stage and have an indolent presentation where fortunately both mother and foetus escape serious harm. However, continued monitoring in the postoperative period would reveal slowly developing symptoms and signs. A high index of suspicion is necessary especially because the foetus is born alive and the mother does not exsanguinate herself. Sometimes I wonder how many patients like this must have escaped notice and intervention and gone home and healed the small rents on their own. It is also possible that such cases that go home with the dehiscence unnoticed after successful vaginal delivery come back after a few days with puerperal sepsis and peritonitis if infection supervened and interfered with the healing as illustrated by a case later.

That brings me to the controversy of whether to explore the scar routinely after delivery. The answer is difficult, and it should be reserved only for cases with excessive bleed or other signs suggestive of scar rupture. Perrotin and colleagues [34] recommended that the exploration of the scar should be done in symptomatic patients only. The Canadian [44] as well as RCOG [36] guidelines also recommend the same.

A defect may feel like a full-thickness defect or a breach of the mucosa and inner layers only, under an intact serosa.

I would like to narrate a few more situations I came across. A woman had a successful VBAC and delivered a healthy luscious baby spontaneously, but had postpartum haemorrhage (PPH). The brisk bleeding compelled an immediate laparotomy. There was full-thickness scar rupture. The right edge of the rupture had involved the uterine artery and hence the brisk bleed. Of course, this patient was managed by suturing the rent, and she consented for sterilization also.

In yet another case, the woman delivered uneventfully. The bleeding appeared slightly excessive. Scar was explored and a rent suspected. Full bladder abdominal and a transvaginal scan confirmed the diagnosis. There was a discontinuity of the lower segment (Fig. 2.5).

Since the patient was stable and not anaemic, she was managed conservatively with antibiotics and monitoring for any deterioration. She recovered uneventfully and was discharged on the 14th day with the advice for interval sterilization and the need to avoid future pregnancies.

A woman was referred to our hospital on the 3rd postpartum day with a fever. She had a successful vaginal delivery after caesarean section at a nursing home. There was no postpartum haemorrhage. She was discharged home 48 h after

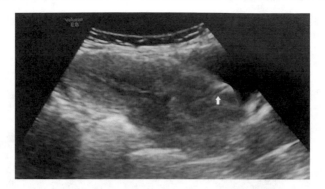

Fig. 2.5   Postpartum sonography confirms discontinuity of scar (*block arrow*)

delivery. At admission the pulse rate was 100/min. There were fever spikes of 101 °F. There were no other localizing symptoms or signs of fever. The abdominal examination revealed mild resistance to palpation, but there were no frank signs of peritonitis. Speculum exam revealed blood-stained minimal discharge and healthy vagina. The uterus was 18-week size. The os was closed, and there was minimal uterine tenderness. She was administered broad-spectrum antibiotics with a working diagnosis of puerperal sepsis. The ultrasound revealed a puerperal uterus and an empty uterine cavity. The uterus was surrounded by minimal free fluid. Blood culture grew *Candida* species, and so parenteral antifungal was administered.

The patient's condition started deteriorating in spite of antibiotics after 48 h with fever spikes persisting and the abdominal fluid collection increasing. She developed tachypnoea and dyspnea, and the oxygen saturation started dropping and so exploratory laparotomy was carried out. There was pus in the peritoneal cavity and full-thickness scar rupture with friable and oedematous margins of the lower segment. The same was repaired. Peritoneal lavage was done, and a drain was inserted. It is possible that the scar must have given way at the second stage without affecting the perinatal outcome. The scar must have got infected due to ascending infection eventually causing peritonitis and deterioration. The woman was not immune-compromised or diabetic. The vagina would have been infected with *Candida* which was not recognized or treated before delivery resulting in such a florid infection of the ruptured scar. A similar case was reported way back in 2005 by Sun and colleagues [46]. However, it was an unscarred uterine dehiscence. She had presented 20 days after the successful vaginal delivery. The authors managed her with laparoscopic repair.

In yet another interesting presentation [32], the woman was found to have omentum protruding from the vagina in the fourth stage of labour after she had a successful VBAC.

Thus, the scar integrity is put to test throughout labour and needs careful monitoring for the various signs alerting a possible dehiscence right from the onset of labour till 48 h or so after delivery.

Box 2.2 summarizes the features that are likely to raise suspicion of scar rupture in the second stage.

Box 2.2 Features of Scar Dehiscence in the Second Stage of Labour
Arrest of descent requiring caesarean section
Arrest of descent requiring instrumental delivery
Foetal heart rates abnormalities
Foetal demise and stillbirth
Cessation of uterine contractions
Bleeding from the vagina in the second stage
Significant postpartum haemorrhage noticed vaginally
Postpartum haemoperitoneum
Postpartum grade III or IV sepsis after VBAC
Haematuria
Suspicion on scar exploration

Though the American and UK College recommend a trial of labour in a woman with previous two caesarean sections, one has to be very cautious. As a policy in our country, we prefer elective caesarean delivery for a woman with previous two caesarean sections. There have been instances where a woman with previous two caesareans came late in labour and delivered uneventfully.

2.3   Rupture Early in Pregnancy in a Scarred Uterus

I would like to narrate the following case. A woman presented in her third pregnancy at 24 weeks of pregnancy in shock. The first delivery was by caesarean section for obstructed labour, and the baby died of birth asphyxia. The second was an elective caesarean section with a good perinatal outcome. In the present pregnancy, there were no other comorbidities. At admission, she was in haemorrhagic shock. The uterine contour was absent, there was haemoperitoneum, and the foetus was dead. There was haematuria. She was resuscitated, and laparotomy revealed a full-thickness scar dehiscence and bladder rent at the dome of the bladder (Fig. 2.6).

The same was repaired, and sterilization was carried out after obtaining informed consent. In this case, the uterus ruptured in the second trimester itself even though the scar had never ruptured in the previous pregnancies. The previous caesarean section was 3 years back. The previous documents showed that the uterus had been closed with a single locking suture due to an adherent urinary bladder that had been drawn up to the lower segment. Inability to achieve double-layer closure and possible high up scar during the previous caesarean could be a possible reason for the extremely weak scar that gave way in the second trimester.

Fig. 2.6 (**a**) Photograph showing ragged rupture of the lower segment in the woman with previous two caesarean sections. (**b**) Urinary bladder rent

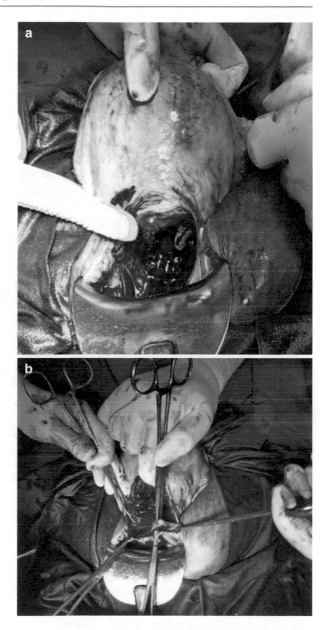

2.4   Scar Ruptures Involving Urinary Bladder

Scar ruptures can sometimes be very complex and difficult involving the urinary bladder. Bladder involvement would substantially increase the morbidity to the mother. It is easy to recognize bladder injury before laparotomy due to the associated haematuria. The primary repair can be very demanding due to the associated friability and the tissue oedema of the bladder wall and surrounding structures.

I have encountered many such referred cases. One such case is of particular interest. She came to the emergency room. Her previous delivery was a caesarean section done in a private nursing home. She complained of vaginal bleed, loss of foetal movements, and diffused pain in the abdomen. She was at 36 weeks of pregnancy and had been in labour for 3 h before presenting to the emergency room. She was pale. There was tachycardia. The systolic blood pressure was 90 mm of Hg. Abdomen showed signs of superficial foetal parts with the loss of contour of the uterus. The foetus was dead. Bladder catheter revealed frank haematuria. The woman was resuscitated. At laparotomy, the foetus and placenta were in the abdominal cavity. After extracting out the baby and placenta, we found that the previous scar had ruptured completely, and the tear had extended downwards towards the vagina on the right side. There was a large linear rent on the posterior wall of the urinary bladder stopping 1 cm short of the ureteric orifice. We had already alerted the urologist. We sutured the lower segment incision. The edges of the downward extension of the lower segment were very oedematous and friable. It was extremely difficult to suture. The extension was closed separate of the lower segment after completely mobilizing the bladder. We used fine catgut sutures to repair as the friable edges were cutting through. The ureteric orifices were visualized. The bladder edges appeared bluish, oedematous, and friable. Layered closure of bladder rent was done with fine sutures. An omental flap was inserted in between the vagina and the bladder. A suprapubic cystotomy was done. The woman was administered broad-spectrum antibiotics. I had thought the sutures will give way, or she will develop a fistula. We continued the bladder drainage for 14 days. Fortunately, she had an uneventful recovery and healed well. Usually, one would encounter bladder involvement transversely on the posterior bladder wall or dome. In the above case, the associated colporrhexis and vertical tear on the posterior bladder wall made it particularly a demanding surgery. Yang [49] observed three cases of the ruptured uterus with bladder injury in a 6-month period. All of them had involved the posterior bladder wall and the anterior wall of the uterus.

Ho and co-authors [24] reported an interesting case that had an uneventful vaginal delivery after caesarean section. They noticed haematuria after the delivery, and it was confirmed to be rupture of the scar involving the posterior bladder wall. If bladder injury is associated with scar dehiscence or rupture, it is very important to follow the principles of tension-free layered closure of the bladder wall. Bladder involvement requires a proper mobilization of the bladder before suturing. The proximity of the tear to the ureteric orifices needs to be looked at in situations with posterior wall or base or bladder involvement. Ureteric catheterization may be necessary if the edge of the tear is very close to the ureteric orifice as there may be kinking of the ureters at the time of double-layer closure. Interposing an omental or peritoneal flap could reduce the risk of fistula formation if the suture lines of the bladder and the lower segment or vagina are very close. Bladder rest in the form of an indwelling catheter for 7 days to sometimes 14 days is necessary depending on the tissue oedema and friability. The indwelling catheter could be urethral or supra-pubic depending on the site of repair and its proximity to the bladder neck.

Some important steps during the primary caesarean could help prevent bladder adhesions and the risk of injury to it if the lower segment ruptures. In this regard following a secondary analysis of cases undergoing repeat caesarean sections, the authors recommend that closure of uterus in two layers is less likely to result in bladder adhesions compared to single-layer closure [7].

2.5   Interesting Cases from Literature and Discussion

The literature has many cases of rupture reported after a caesarean section.

I enumerate a few of the cases listed in the literature below for their extremely rarity and challenging individualized management.

Zhang and colleagues [50] reported an interesting case of asymptomatic large full-thickness defect in the lower uterine segment at repeat caesarean section in a woman who had undergone uterine packing to control haemorrhage at previous caesarean section.

Ahmadi and co-authors [2] reported an extremely interesting case of scar dehiscence noticed in a patient with previous caesarean section at 24 weeks of pregnancy which was managed conservatively till 34 weeks when repeat caesar-ean section was performed to deliver a live baby. The woman had complained of pain in the abdomen, and the dehiscence with amniotic sac bulging was diagnosed on the scan. The foetus was doing well. As she was stable and was very keen to continue the pregnancy, the decision for conservative management was taken after discussion and counselling with the woman and her husband. The decision was collectively taken by the couple and the medical team after understanding the pos-sible risks. One-to-one intense monitoring was carried out after admission in the unit.

A similar case has been reported by other authors [21, 33]. In the latter case, the woman was conservatively managed till 33 weeks on an outpatient basis, though the defect had been diagnosed at 17 weeks of pregnancy. It is interesting to note that in spite of an obvious full-thickness defect, the pregnancy was continued till the foetus was mature enough to be salvaged by elective caesarean resulting in a favourable outcome.

Stitely and co-authors [45] reported a woman with previous caesarean section. She was planned for surgical termination of pregnancy at 13 weeks of gestation. She developed scar dehiscence when preoperative priming of the cervix was carried out with misoprostol.

Recently Bolla and colleagues [8] reported a pregnant woman with previous cae-sarean section who was found to have a scar dehiscence at 8 weeks of gestation. The authors sutured the same by laparoscopy, and elective caesarean section was carried out later at 38 weeks. These above situations are rare when the scar dehiscence is not associated with maternal compromise and foetal jeopardy. Suturing and con-tinuation till term could be a possible alternative.

There is a rise in the number of previous caesarean pregnancies. It is therefore very essential to identify the factors which might result in a weak scar that might give way during labour. Extensive research has been done to predict scar dehiscence in a woman undergoing a trial of labour.

Guise et al. [20] undertook a review of various studies that included pregnant women after one caesarean section. They shortlisted 203 studies. They found that the risk of scar rupture after a caesarean was 3 per 1000. The risk was 4.7/1000 in women planned for the trial of labour, and it was 0.26 per 1000 in elective repeat caesarean section.

Al-Zirqi et al. [4] observed a rate of rupture of a total of 2/1000 for the pre-labour caesarean section. It was the lowest (0.7 %) for women who had elective repeat caesarean section, and the rupture was found to be significantly higher at 6.7/1000 among women who had a trial of labour. They further observed that among the 80 women who had rupture after the trial of labour, five were after spontaneous vaginal delivery and five had vacuum delivery. Age above 40 years, failed trial of labour, unplanned emergency pre-labour caesarean section, induction of labour, and gestational age at or above 41 weeks were found to be factors that significantly increased the risk of rupture.

In a 1-year case-control study from the UK [18], the risk of uterine rupture was found to be 0.2 per 1000 maternities overall and 2.1 and 0.3 per 1000 maternities in women with a previous caesarean delivery planning vaginal or elective caesarean delivery, respectively. The risk increased three times in women with previous two caesarean sections and those with interpregnancy interval shorter than 12 months since their last caesarean delivery. Labour induction and oxytocin use increased the risk by four times. They observed a case fatality rate of 1.3 % and 124 per 1000 perinatal mortality.

Kok et al. [26] conducted a prospective cohort analysis from Dutch perinatal registry. They studied the risk of rupture among women delivering after a previously planned caesarean section and compared it with women delivering after a previous emergency caesarean section. The risk of scar rupture during a trial of labour in a subsequent pregnancy after previously planned elective caesarean was significantly higher (OR 1.6) at 0.3 % compared to 0.2 % in those who had a previous emergency caesarean. In the group who underwent elective repeat caesarean also, the incidental finding of scar dehiscence was higher (0.07 %) in those who had a previously planned caesarean compared to 0.04 % among those who had a previous emergency caesarean section.

Thus, the presence of labour before a caesarean section gives a stronger scar subsequently probably because labour helps to identify the lower segment better and gives a scope of double-layer closure with a better formed lower segment.

In a 7-year review of the cases in a large tertiary institute in India by Sinha et al. [42], the authors found the incidence of rupture to be 0.318 % in women with a history of prior uterine surgery and to be 0.02 % in women without a history of any prior uterine surgery. Among the 47 cases of rupture, 14 did not have any scar, and all these cases were in labour. 24 out of the 33 cases of rupture of scarred uterus had a low transverse caesarean scar. Among these 24 cases, labour was induced in 9, 4 were not in labour, and 11 had spontaneous labour.

One has to be very prudent in selecting the cases with previous caesarean section for allowing for vaginal delivery. Various factors affect the healing of the uterine incision like the previous indication, the interval from the last childbirth, the intra-operative details including the extension of the uterine incision, the type of uterine incision, the type of closure of the uterine incision, and the postoperative infection of the uterine incision. Certain factors in the ongoing pregnancy like the estimated weight of the foetus and the adequacy of the pelvis for the foetus also influence the decision for TOLAC.

One must follow the guidelines (RCOG revised in 2015) before planning TOLAC in a woman with previous caesarean section. The risk of dehiscence of a previous low transverse caesarean scar is 0.2–0.7 % which increases to 2–9 % if the previous scar involved the upper segment (classical/J-shaped extension). The risk increases by two- to threefold when the inter-delivery interval is 12–24 months (RCOG 2015) [36].

Veena et al. [48] carried out a retrospective study in a referral Institute of South India over a 2-year period. They observed 93 cases in the period studied. The incidence of ruptured uterus was 0.28 %. 95 % were multiparous, and more than three-fourths of the cases with rupture were in women with a previous caesarean scar. Sixty-four percent of women with a previous caesarean had interpregnancy interval of <18 months' duration from the last caesarean section. Fifty percent of ruptures in previous caesarean cases were following the trial of labour. Seven (all without scars) out of the 93 women with rupture had undergone induction of labour.

In a recent study, Brahmalakshmy and Kushtagi [9] analysed the obstetric and non-obstetric variables among women undergoing repeat elective caesarean section and correlated the intraoperative scar grade with the various factors. They observed that primary caesarean performed before term, single-layer closure, and a shorter than 54 months interpregnancy interval were significantly associated with thinner scars. Further age more than 35 years, prolonged rupture of membranes more than 18 h and baby weight more than 3 kg at the primary caesarean, and postpartum fever were also associated with thin scar though it was not statistically significant.

Sevket et al. [40] conducted a randomized trial of women undergoing elective caesarean. They randomly assigned them to the closure of caesarean incision with either single layer or double layer. The authors demonstrated that the healing ratio and the myometrium covering the scar (the measures of uterine scar healing) at 6 months as measured by hydrosonography were significantly higher in those who underwent closure by double layer versus those by a single layer.

In a study by Micek et al. [30], previous vaginal delivery (either VBAC or otherwise) and spontaneous onset of labour were found to be the most important factor predicting successful VBAC. Similar findings were observed by other authors [28].

Based on the observations of a case (successful VBAC)-control (failed VBAC) study [6], the authors concluded that a previous history of vaginal delivery after the caesarean, spontaneous rupture of membranes with labour, and a cervix more than 3 cm at admission are associated with higher chances of successful vaginal delivery. They further observed that meconium staining of liquor, malposition, and history of stillbirth are more likely to be associated with failed VBAC. These authors did not find factors like inter-delivery interval, maternal age, the indication of the previous caesarean, and the birth weight to be significant determinants of successful VBAC.

The risk of rupture increases many times when labour is induced or augmented compared to the spontaneous onset of labour. Dekker et al.[15] conducted a population-based retrospective cohort study and observed a three- to fivefold increased risk of rupture for any induction and sixfold increased risk for prostaglandin combined with oxytocin, and the risk of rupture was highest at 14-fold for augmentation with oxytocin. The risk of rupture goes up many times when prostaglandins are used for induction compared to mechanical methods of induction. The serious perinatal outcomes increased by 41-fold in ruptures after induction of labour and by 15-fold in ruptures after spontaneous labour among women with previous caesarean scars [3]. The reason being the need for augmentation is likely when the labour has become protracted after achieving active labour which is an indirect warning about likely dehiscence or underlying disproportion.

Bujold et al. [10] conducted a case-control study with 1:3 ratio of the case (previous caesarean in labour who had rupture) with the control (previous caesarean in labour who did not rupture). They observed that the risk of rupture increases significantly with single-layer closure (OR = 2.69) and birth weight more than 3.5 kg (OR = 2.03).

In a meta-analysis of various studies, Roberge et al.[37] reviewed nine studies that included a total of 5810 women undergoing trial after previous caesarean section and concluded that previous closure with locked single-layer had five times higher risk of rupture compared to double-layer closure. The risk was not increased with non-locked single-layer closure of the previous caesarean when compared to previous double-layer closure.

However, in a retrospective comparative study, Hudic and colleagues [25] did not find any significant difference in the rate of ruptures among women with previous locked versus unlocked single-layer closure.

Scientists have looked at the scar thickness a week before delivery and have used various cutoffs to predict dehiscence.

Sharma et al. [41] studied a hundred women with or without previous caesarean and observed that the sonographic thickness of the scar was significantly less in women with previous caesarean sections.

Bujold and co-authors [11] conducted a prospective cohort study and recommended a cutoff value of 2.3 mm for scar thickness. The risk of rupture is very high if the scar is thinner than this and should preclude trial of labour.

Mohammed et al. [31] conducted a prospective controlled study on pregnant women. They had three groups: one group of patients with previous one caesarean, another group who had previous VBAC, and the third who had unscarred controls. They studied the scar thickness by the transabdominal and vaginal scan. The scar dehiscence rate was found to be 28%, and it occurred only in the group without previous VBAC. The dehiscence was significantly more in women in whom the first caesarean section was performed for cephalopelvic disproportion and when the interpregnancy interval was short. The authors observed that a scar thinner than 2.5 mm on scan had a higher risk of rupture.

Vaginal and abdominal scans are recommended for measuring the lower uterine segment thickness. However, Laflammo et al. [27] reported two cases who had the previous caesarean performed at 29 weeks. In the subsequent pregnancy, the vaginal scan missed a scar dehiscence which was high up on the lower segment that was picked up on abdominal scan only. So it may be prudent to use both routes of the scan in patients to double check for the entire lower segment.

Uharček and colleagues [47] recommend a cutoff of 2.5 mm as the scar thickness for a sensitivity of 90.9 % and negative predictive value of 95.5 %.

Recently Mansour and colleagues [29] have recommended multiplanar view 3D scan for assessment of scar dehiscence before labour, and they found it to have nearly 100 % specificity and positive predictive value.

A few authors [39, 43] have tried to work out a prediction model for the possibility of rupture in the subsequent pregnancies based on the adjusted log likelihood ratio. An admission scoring system was designed by Flamm and Geiger [19]. Evidence-based patient decision aid in the form of a booklet has been developed recently [38].

High-Risk Factors for Intrapartum Scar Dehiscence
Age >40 years
Birth interval <18 months
Previous classical caesarean
Previous PT caesarean
Previous caesarean for placenta previa
Previous extension of uterine incision
Previous uterine wound infection
Expected birth weight more than 3.5 kg in the index pregnancy
Scar thickness less than 2.5 mm
Previous uterine closure with single layer locked
Induction/augmentation with oxytocin
Induction with prostaglandins

Randomized control trials would be the ideal way to study the risk of rupture with the type of closure, the number of layers of closure, and the sutures used at the closure.

The CAESER and CORONIS trials [12, 14] have shown that for various parameters like blunt versus sharp dissection, single-/double-layer closure, catgut versus polyglactin, and closure versus non-closure of the peritoneum, the short-term outcomes are comparable. The results for the long-term outcomes including the risk of rupture in subsequent pregnancies during labour are yet awaited.

Thus to summarize the scar rupture can occur silently without labour. It can occur anytime during labour including the second stage of labour. It may sometimes get recognized after delivery. The following table summarizes the rare or atypical presentations of scar rupture.

Rare Presentation
Scar dehiscence on routine scan in antenatal period
Abdominal pain anytime during pregnancy
Shock in early pregnancy in a previous scarred uterus
Antepartum haemorrhage
Postpartum haemorrhage
Postpartum peritonism and haemoperitoneum
Puerperal sepsis grade 3 or 4

References

1. ACOG Practice bulletin no. 115. Vaginal birth after previous cesarean delivery. Obstet Gynecol. 2010;116(2 Pt 1):450–63.
2. Ahmadi F, Shiva S, Akhbari F. Incomplete cesarean scar rupture. J Reprod Infertil. 2013;14(1):43–5.
3. Al-Zirqi I, Stray-Pedersen B, Forsen L, et al. Uterine rupture after previous caesarean section. BJOG. 2010;117(7):809–20. doi:10.1111/j.1471-0528.2010.02533.x.Epub2010M.
4. Al-Zirqi I, Stray-Pedersen B, Forsén L, Daltveit AK, Vangen S. Uterine rupture: trends over 40 years. BJOG. 2015;123(5):780–7. doi:10.1111/1471-0528.13394 [Epub ahead of print].
5. Andersen MM, Thisted DL, Amer-Wåhlin I, Krebs L, Danish CTG, Monitoring during VBAC study group. Can intrapartum cardiotocography predict uterine rupture among women with prior caesarean delivery?: a population-based case-control study. PLoS One. 2016;11(2):e0146347. doi:10.1371/journal.pone.0146347. eCollection 2016.
6. Birara M, Gebrehiwot Y. Factors associated with the success of vaginal birth after one caesarean section (VBAC) at three teaching hospitals in Addis Ababa, Ethiopia: a case control study. BMC Pregnancy Childb. 2013;13:31. doi:10.1186/1471-2393-13-31.
7. Blumenfeld YJ, Caughey AB, El-Sayed YY, Daniels K, Lyell DJ. Single- versus double-layer hysterotomy closure at primary caesarean delivery and bladder adhesions. BJOG. 2010;117(6):690–4. doi:10.1111/j.1471-0528.2010.02529.x. Epub 2010 Mar 12.
8. Bolla D, Raio L, Favre D, Papadia A, In-Albon S, Mueller MD. Laparoscopic ultrasound-guided repair of uterine scar isthmocele connected with the extra-amniotic space in early pregnancy. J Minim Invasive Gynecol. 2016;23(2):261–4. doi:10.1016/j.jmig.2015.09.010. Epub 2015 Sep 25.
9. Brahmalakshmy BL, Kushtagi P. Variables influencing the integrity of lower uterine segment in post-cesarean pregnancy. Arch Gynecol Obstet. 2015;291(4):755–62. doi:10.1007/s00404-014-3455-6. Epub 2014 Sep 11.
10. Bujold E, Goyet M, Marcoux S, Brassard N, Cormier B, Hamilton E, Abdous B, Sidi EA, Kinch R, Miner L, Masse A, Fortin C, Gagné GP, Fortier A, Bastien G, Sabbah R, Guimond P, Roberge S, Gauthier RJ. The role of uterine closure in the risk of uterine rupture. Obstet Gynecol. 2010;116(1):43–50. doi:10.1097/AOG.0b013e3181e41be3.
11. Bujold E, Jastrow N, Simoneau J, Brunet S, Gauthier RJ. Prediction of complete uterine rupture by sonographic evaluation of the lower uterine segment. Am J Obstet Gynecol. 2009;201(3):320. doi:10.1016/j.ajog.2009.06.014.e1-6.

12. CAESAR study collaborative group. Caesarean section surgical techniques: a randomised factorial trial (CAESAR). BJOG. 2010;117(11):1366–76. doi:10.1111/j.1471-0528.2010.02686.x.
13. Cohen A, Cohen Y, Laskov I, Maslovitz S, Lessing JB, Many A. Persistent abdominal pain over uterine scar during labor as a predictor of delivery complications. Int J Gynaecol Obstet. 2013;123(3):200–2. doi:10.1016/j.ijgo.2013.06.018. Epub 2013 Aug 31.
14. The CORONIS Collaborative Group. CORONIS – the International study of caesarean section surgical techniques: the follow-up study. BMC Pregnancy Childbirth. 2013;13:215. doi:10.1186/1471-2393-13-215. Published online 2013 Nov 21.
15. Dekker GA, Chan A, Luke CG, Priest K, Riley M, Halliday J, King JF, Gee V, O'Neill M, Snell M, Cull V, Cornes S. Risk of uterine rupture in Australian women attempting vaginal birth after one prior caesarean section: a retrospective population-based cohort study. BJOG. 2010;117(11):1358–65. doi:10.1111/j.1471-0528.2010.02688.x. Epub 2010 Aug 17.
16. Desseauve D, Bonifazi-Grenouilleau M, Fritel X, Lathélize J, Sarreau M, Pierre F. Fetal heart rate abnormalities associated with uterine rupture: a case-control study: a new time-lapse approach using a standardized classification. Eur J Obstet Gynecol Reprod Biol. 2016;197:16–21. doi:10.1016/j.ejogrb.2015.10.019. Epub 2015 Dec 2.
17. FIGO consensus guidelines on intrapartum fetal monitoring: cardiotocography (October 2015) http://www.figo.org/news/available-view-figo-intrapartum-fetal-monitoring-guidelines-0015088. Accessed on 16 Apr 2016.
18. Fitzpatrick KE, Kurinczuk JJ, Alfirevic Z, Spark P, Brocklehurst P, Knight M. Uterine rupture by intended mode of delivery in the UK: a national case-control study. PLoS Med. 2012;9(3):e1001184. doi:10.1371/journal.pmed.1001184. Epub 2012 Mar 13.
19. Flamm BL, Geiger AM. Vaginal birth after cesarean delivery: an admission scoring system. Obstet Gynecol. 1997;90:907.
20. Guise J-M, Eden K, Emeis C, Denman MA, Marshall N, Fu R, Janik R, Nygren P, Walker M, McDonagh M. Vaginal Birth After Cesarean: New Insights. Evidence Report/Technology Assessment No.191. (Prepared by the Oregon Health & Science University Evidence-based Practice Center under Contract No. 290-2007-10057-I). AHRQ Publication No. 10-E003. Rockville, MD: Agency for Healthcare Research and Quality. March 2010.
21. Hamar BD, Levine D, Katz NL, Lim KH. Expectant management of uterine dehiscence in the second trimester of pregnancy. Obstet Gynecol. 2003;102:1139–42.
22. Haresh UD, Rohit KJ, Aarti AV. Prognostic factors for successful vaginal birth after cesarean section – analysis of 162 cases. J Obstet Gynaecol India. 2010;60(6):498–502.
23. Harper LM, Cahill AG, Roehl KA, Odibo AO, Stamilio DM, Macones GA. The pattern of labor preceding uterine rupture. Am J Obstet Gynecol. 2012;207(3):210. e1-6.
24. Ho SY, Chang SD, Liang CC. Simultaneous uterine and urinary bladder rupture in an otherwise successful vaginal birth after cesarean delivery. J Chin Med Assoc. 2010;73(12):655–9. doi:10.1016/S1726-4901(10)70143-X.
25. Hudic I, Bujold E, Fatusic Z, Roberge S, Mandzic A, Fatusic J. Risk of uterine rupture following locked vs unlocked single-layer closure. Med Arch. 2012;66(6):412–4.
26. Kok N, Ruiter L, Hof M, Ravelli A, Mol BW, Pajkrt E, Kazemier B. Risk of maternal and neonatal complications in a subsequent pregnancy after planned caesarean section in a first birth, compared with emergency caesarean section: a nationwide comparative cohort study. BJOG. 2014;121(2):216–23. doi:10.1111/1471-0528.12483.
27. Laflamme SM, Jastrow N, Girard M, Paris G, Bérubé L, Bujold E. Pitfall in ultrasound evaluation of uterine scar from prior preterm cesarean section. AJP Rep. 2011;1(1):65–8. doi:10.10 55/s-0031-1284222. Epub 2011 Jul 22.
28. Madaan M, Agrawal S, Nigam A, Aggarwal R, Trivedi SS. Trial of labour after previous caesarean section: the predictive factors affecting the outcome. J Obstet Gynaecol. 2011;31(3):224–8. doi:10.3109/01443615.2010.544426.
29. Mansour GM, El-Mekkawi SF, Khairy HT, Mossad AE. Feasibility of prediction of cesarean section scar dehiscence in the third trimester by three-dimensional ultrasound. J Matern Fetal Neonatal Med. 2015;28(8):944–8.

30. Micek M, Kosinska-Kaczynska K, Godek B, Krowicka M, Szymusik I, Wielgos M. Birth after a previous cesarean section – what is most important in making a decision? Neuro Endocrinol Lett. 2014;35(8):718–23.
31. Mohammed AB, Al-Moghazi DA, Hamdy MT, Mohammed EM. Ultrasonographic evaluation of lower uterine segment thickness in pregnant women with previous cesarean section. Middle East Fertil Soc J. 2010;15(3):188–93. doi:10.1016/j.mefs.2010.06.006.
32. Mwenda AS. 4th stage transvaginal omental herniation during VBAC complicated by shoulder dystocia: a unique presentation of uterine rupture. BMC Pregnancy Childbirth. 2013;13:76 (ISSN: 1471-2393).
33. Oyelese Y, Tchabo JG, Chapin B, Nair A, Hanson P, McLaren R. Conservative management of uterine rupture diagnosed prenatally on the basis of sonography. J Ultrasound Med. 2003;22:977–80.
34. Perrotin F, Marret H, Fignon A, Body G, Lansac J. Scarred uterus: is a routine exploration of the cesarean scar after vaginal birth always necessary? [Article in French]. J Gynecol Obstet Biol Reprod (Paris). 1999;28(3):253–62.
35. Qureshi B, Inafuku K, Oshima K, Masamoto H, Kanazawa K. Ultrasonographic evaluation of lower uterine segment to predict the integrity and quality of cesarean scar during pregnancy: a prospective study. Tohoku J Exp Med. 1997;183(1):55–65.
36. RCOG guidelines Birth after Previous Caesarean Birth (Green-top Guideline No. 45) Published: 01/10/2015 https://www.rcog.org.uk/en/guidelines-research-services/guidelines/gtg45/. Accessed on 16 Apr 2016.
37. Roberge S, Chaillet N, Boutin A, Moore L, Jastrow N, Brassard N, Gauthier RJ, Hudic I, Shipp TD, Weimar CH, Fatusic Z, Demers S, Bujold E. Single- versus double-layer closure of the hysterotomy incision during cesarean delivery and risk of uterine rupture. Int J Gynaecol Obstet. 2011;115(1):5–10. doi:10.1016/j.ijgo.2011.04.013. Epub 2011 Jul 26.
38. Schoorel EN, van Kuijk SM, Melman S, et al. Vaginal birth after a caesarean section: the development of a Western European population-based prediction model for deliveries at term. BJOG. 2014;121(2):194–201. doi:10.1111/1471-0528.12539; discussion 201.
39. Scifres CM, Rohn A, Odibo A, Stamilio D, Macones GA. Predicting significant maternal morbidity in women attempting vaginal birth after cesarean section. Am J Perinatol. 2011;28(3):181–6. doi:10.1055/s-0030-1266159. Epub 2010 Sep 14.
40. Sevket O, Ates S, Molla T, Ozkal F, Uysal O, Dansuk R. Hydrosonographic assessment of the effects of 2 different suturing techniques on the healing of the uterine scar after cesarean delivery. Int J Gynaecol Obstet. 2014;125(3):219–22. doi:10.1016/j.ijgo.2013.11.013. Epub 2014 Feb 28.
41. Sharma C, Surya M, Soni A, Soni P, Verma A, Verma S. Sonographic prediction of scar dehiscence in women with previous cesarean section. J Obstet Gynaecol India. 2015;65(2):97–103. doi:10.1007/s13224-014-0630-4. Epub 2014 Nov 4.
42. Sinha M, Gupta R, Gupta P, Rani R, Kaur R, Singh R. Uterine rupture: a seven year review at a tertiary care hospital in New Delhi, India. Indian J Community Med. 2016;41(1):45–9. doi:10.4103/0970-0218.170966.
43. Smith GC, White IR, Pell JP, Dobbie R. Predicting cesarean section and uterine rupture among women attempting vaginal birth after prior cesarean section. PLoS Med. 2005;2(9):e252. Epub 2005 Sep 13.
44. SOGC Clinical Practice Guidelines. Guidelines for vaginal birth after previous Caesarean birth. No 155 (Replaces guideline No 147), February 2005. http://sogc.org/wp-content/uploads/2013/01/155E-CPG-February2005.pdf 10.3109/14767058.2014.938626. Epub 2014 Jul 22. Accessed 16 Mar 2016.
45. Stitely ML, Craw S, Africano E, Reid R. Uterine scar dehiscence associated with misoprostol cervical priming for surgical abortion: a case report. J Reprod Med. 2015;60(9–10):445–8.
46. Sun CH, Liao CI, Kan YY. "Silent" rupture of the unscarred gravid uterus with subsequent pelvic abscess: successful laparoscopic management. J Minim Invasive Gynecol. 2005;12(6):519–21.

47. Uharček P, Brešťanský A, Ravinger J, Máňová A, Zajacová M. Sonographic assessment of lower uterine segment thickness at term in women with previous cesarean delivery. Arch Gynecol Obstet. 2015;292(3):609–12. doi:10.1007/s00404-015-3687-0. Epub 2015 Mar 27.
48. Veena P, Habeebullah S, Chaturvedula A. A review of 93 cases of ruptured uterus over a period of 2 years in a tertiary care hospital in South India. J Obstet Gynaecol. 2012;32(3):260–3. doi :10.3109/01443615.2011.638091.
49. Yang B. Bladder rupture associated with uterine rupture at delivery. Int Urogynecol J. 2011;22(5):625–7. doi:10.1007/s00192-010-1318-7. Epub 2010 Nov 25.
50. Zhang J, Chen SF, Luo YE. Asymptomatic spontaneous complete uterine rupture in a term pregnancy after uterine packing during previous caesarean section: a case report. Clin Exp Obstet Gynecol. 2014;41(5):597–8.

Rupture of Apparently Unscarred Uterus

3

There have been many occasions when a multigravida with neglected labour presented to the emergency room in shock with the clinical features of tachycardia (low volume pulse), hypotension, and severe pallor. The woman may not complain of much pain because the violent contractions have ceased. In a typical case, the abdominal examination would reveal free fluid (haemoperitoneum), superficial foetal parts, absent foetal heart sounds, and variable (usually mild) vaginal bleed. Vaginal examination in such a scenario would reveal recession of the presenting part or no foetal parts felt either through the os if it admits a finger or through the fornices.

Developed countries have phased out rupture of the uterus due to neglected and obstructed labour. Unfortunately, these maladies still happen in our and other developing countries [11–13]. These have distinctly come down over the last two decades with efficient referrals and emergency obstetric facilities made available at community health centres. It was very disheartening to read the article by Prajapati and co-authors [10]. The authors reported three cases on whom they performed a postmortem. All of them were reported to have difficult labour, and postmortem revealed haemorrhagic shock with ruptured uterus and foetus in the peritoneal cavity.

Such cases should be recognized early, and one must carry out the needful like resuscitation and definitive treatment with laparotomy promptly. If recognized early and treated appropriately, the maternal mortality due to ruptured uterus and haemorrhagic shock should be brought to zero.

Singh and Shrivastava [13] reported rate of rupture of 0.152 % in women without a uterine scar. In yet another study from Rohtak (North of India), Gupta and Nanda [7] reported that 52.6 % cases of rupture were due to neglect and obstructed labour.

Khooharo et al. [8] observed that the incidence of ruptured uterus was 20 % in obstructed labour. They studied 40 patients with obstructed labour and barring one woman who was a primigravida, all the other seven women who ruptured their uterus were multigravida. Rupture of the uterus following obstructed labour has high perinatal mortality. Fortunately, this kind of a typical case is very easy to recognize even by an undergraduate student.

© Springer Nature Singapore Pte Ltd. 2017

G. Dorairajan, *Ruptured Uterus*, DOI 10.1007/978-981-10-2852-6_3

However, a rupture of the uterus in a multigravida can have varied presentations.

3.1 Rupture in the Second Stage

I would like to narrate a few cases. A woman pregnant for the second time with a previous normal, uneventful delivery presented in labour. I examined her at admission. The vitals were normal. She was not anaemic. Abdomen revealed a singleton term foetus with moderate contractions. The foetal heart sound was 120 dropping to 100/min. On vaginal examination, she was fully dilated with vertex at +2 station and a normal pelvis. There was no caput or moulding. I admitted her and informed the sister to take her delivery immediately. The dropping foetal heart sound worried me. I got a call from the sister half an hour later that she has not delivered, and the foetal heart sound is no longer heard. I rushed to attend to her. She was stable. Pulse was 100/min. BP was 120/70 mm of Hg. There were no contractions, and the foetal heart sound was absent. On vaginal examination, the head had receded to 0 station. There was no bleeding from the vagina. When I inserted a urinary catheter, there was frank haematuria. I wheeled her for immediate laparotomy which confirmed a rent in the left lateral wall (Fig. 3.1) involving both the upper and lower segments. The rent had

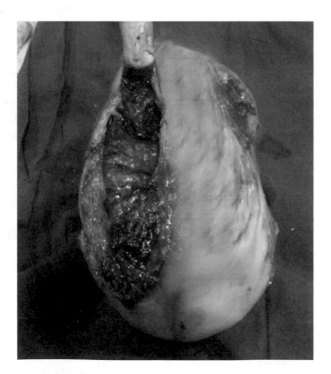

Fig. 3.1 Rupture of the lateral wall of the uterus

involved the bladder, and the foetus was lying in the peritoneal cavity. I had to resort to a hysterectomy. The bladder rent was repaired.

Unlike the bladder rents following obstructed labour or involving previous scars, in this case, the edges of the bladder rent did not seem to be oedematous or friable. On later questioning, she gave a history of curettage for a previous spontaneous abortion. I presume there must have been a low perforation with the bladder getting adhered to it. It is very important to understand that the uterus is likely to rupture in the second stage after going through the whole labour if there is a weak point in the lower segment. Xia and colleagues [20] reported two cases, one of whom had a scarring due to placenta accreta and the other without apparent cause. Both these cases also had manifested with foetal bradycardia before manifesting rupture. Foetal heart rate abnormalities were found to be the most frequent manifestation [6] among the 25 cases with complete rupture in a retrospective analysis of ruptures over 20 years. The gradual diminution of amplitude of uterine contraction followed by severe prolonged bradycardia has been described as staircase sign by Matsuo and colleagues [9].

The case emphasizes the need to monitor and be vigilant even in the second stage of a woman who appears to be a low-risk case in labour.

I would like to detail another case I had managed about 10 years back. The case was handed over to me in the labour room as a third gravida with previous two normal deliveries. She had been admitted half an hour earlier with term pregnancy in the second stage with foetal demise. There was no history of bleeding. She had been started on oxytocin drip as there had been no contractions observed at admission. When I examined the woman, she appeared peaceful and comfortable. Her pulse was 90/min. Blood pressure was 120/80 mm of Hg. She was mildly anaemic. Abdominal examination revealed term size uterus with expected foetal weight of 3 kg. The contour was well made out. There were no contractions. The foetal heart sound was absent. Vaginal examination revealed a fully dilated and effaced cervix. The vertex was at 0 station. There was no caput or moulding. There was no bleeding. The pelvis was normal gynaecoid. She did not have any pain. In fact, she requested me to do a caesarean as she had not delivered in spite of 1 h of being in the second stage. I reassured her and counselled for oxytocin drip and vaginal delivery. I continued the oxytocin drip. The patient's condition remained the same. The labour had come to a standstill. Contractions failed to establish, so I took her up for a caesarean section as she refused any destructive operation. On opening the abdomen, I observed that the lower segment had completely given way with the shoulders presenting at the edges of the rupture. The foetal trunk and breech were still inside the upper segment. There was minimal haemoperitoneum. The shoulders had probably tamponade the ruptured edges (Fig. 3.2).

It indeed made me feel miserable to have missed rupture. In this case, foetal demise and the loss of uterine contractions in established labour especially in the second stage were the features signalling possible rupture. In the previously discussed case, the sequence of events happened right after admission, and the changing findings with the contractions ceasing, the station receding, and the foetal heart disappearing were clear features of rupture. Thus even though the woman is stable without any other features of rupture, these two important findings of cessation of

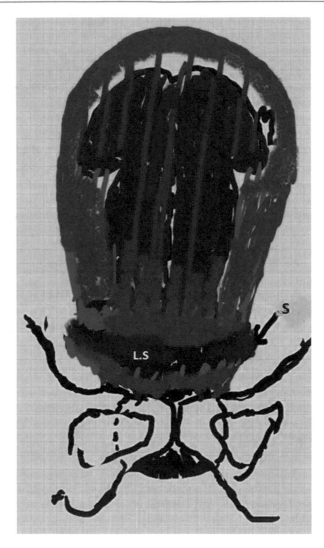

Fig. 3.2 Line diagram depicting tamponade by shoulders *s* on the edges of the ruptured lower segment *LS* preventing exsanguination

contractions and foetal demise in labour in a multigravid woman may be the only clue for suspecting rupture especially when the previous record of the station of the presenting part is not available. I still vividly remember the name and face of the patient and her earnest request for caesarean. Fortunately, I did not try any instrumentation or destructive procedure. The adage that when a multiparous woman feels that something is not well with her in established labour, we need to heed to her, is so true for this case. There was no other cause for this rupture other than the fact that she was a multiparous woman.

3.2   Rupture Misdiagnosed as Antepartum Haemorrhage Due to Placenta Previa

I would like to narrate two cases that bring out a close differential diagnosis confusing the picture and delaying the diagnosis.

A woman in her third pregnancy presented at term pregnancy with bleeding from the vagina. It was the first episode of bleeding. She was in shock at admission. Abdominal examination, however, revealed a lax abdominal wall with a poor tone of the rectus muscle. The contour was made out. The foetal parts were not superficially palpable but were easily palpable. There were no uterine contractions. The duty resident made a diagnosis of placenta previa with intrauterine foetal demise. The patient was quickly resuscitated and wheeled for caesarean. At laparotomy it was realized that the uterus had ruptured, the foetus was in the amniotic sac with fluid pockets around it, and the back of the foetus was under the abdominal wall resulting in a false sign of maintained contour of the uterus. What was perceived as low-lying placenta on sonography was the retracted uterus. In this case, the definitive management was immediate laparotomy as she was in shock. So the exact preoperative diagnosis may be inconsequential.

I would like to narrate yet another interesting case we recently managed in our hospital. A woman pregnant for the third time, with previous two normal deliveries, was referred from a primary health centre as a case of suspected abruption. She was 32 weeks pregnant and complained of sudden onset painful bleeding followed by loss of foetal movements. She was not hypertensive. There was no history of trauma or previous fibroids. She had been transfused a pint of blood in the primary health centre 16 h before she came to our hospital. Her pregnancy was so far unsupervised. There was no history of prior caesarean/abortions/uterine procedures.

At admission to our hospital, her pulse was 100/min and blood pressure was 110/70 mm of Hg. She was moderately pale, ill-nourished, and asthenic. The admitting resident made a diagnosis of abruption because the uterus was 32 weeks size with normal contour and slight tenderness. The foetal heart sound was absent. The cervix was uneffaced and closed, and there was no bleeding observed. Urinary catheter revealed high-coloured but adequate urine. We transfused one more pint of whole blood as the baseline investigations revealed moderate anaemia with a haemoglobin of 6.5 g%. The coagulation profile and blood urea and creatinine were normal. Labour induction was started with 50 μg of misoprostol sublingually. The junior consultant reviewed the case and concurred with the clinical findings. The bedside sonography by the consultant revealed a foetus with signs of spalding, with adequate liquor around the foetus. The foetus was presenting as vertex high up. The placenta was found anterior, but a succenturiate lobe of the placenta was found to be overlying the os. There was no free fluid. The revised diagnosis was as placenta previa with foetal demise. The patient had not responded to labour induction. The case was discussed with me and I saw the woman nearly 36 h after admission. I observed that she was asthenic, ill-nourished, and not in pain. Her pulse had settled to 90/min. and BP was stable at 120/80. There was adequate urine output. Abdominal examination revealed a 32-week size relaxed uterus with absent foetal heart sounds. Vaginal examination revealed a closed cervix but no presenting part from the fornices. We discussed, and since she was stable with a macerated foetus, with placenta previa, with no further bleed, we took a calculated risk of extra-amniotic saline instillation after counselling and discussing with the woman. The same was performed uneventfully. She was under strict observation for any bleeding. Facilities for immediate caesarean section were kept ready in the case of bleeding. She remained status quo for the next 24 h. I must confess I was internally reflecting with the finding of no presenting part from the fornices gnawing at me, when in the middle of the night I woke up agonized when it dawned on me that we have missed ruptured uterus. I felt miserable. Laparotomy confirmed a longitudinal rupture of the anterior wall of the upper segment (Fig. 3.3).

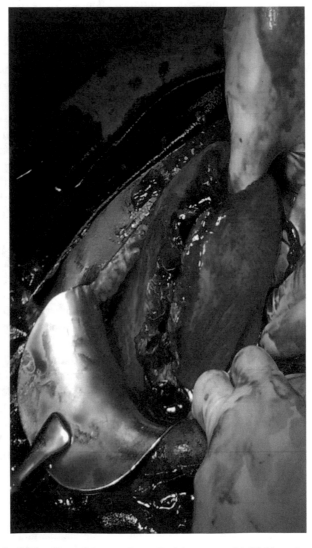

Fig. 3.3 Longitudinal rupture of the anterior wall of the uterus with friable oedematous margins

The foetus was lying in the peritoneal cavity with intact membranes and amniotic fluid. The placenta was anterior and so was the back of the foetus. There was about 400 ml haemoperitoneum.

The case humbled me. Thinking back, I realized that the bias of admission diagnosis, the false appearance of preserved contour due to anterior back with intact amniotic sac and amniotic fluid around it, and the steadily settling pulse rate and stable blood pressure had misled me.

However, there were enough typical features. The presence of painful bleeding, moderate pallor, and inability to establish labour with inducing agents and the lack of presenting part from the fornices or through the cervical os are glaring enough to suggest rupture. The woman was not in shock possibly due to retraction of the uterine margins which were no longer bleeding briskly inside. These cases may get misdiagnosed as antepartum haemorrhage due to low-lying placenta or abruption placenta at the first presentation.

I would like to bring out this important take-home message and an important component of the checklist. I would like to emphasize that whenever one does an abdominal sonography for cases of antepartum haemorrhage, one should look at the continuity of the uterus from the cervix preferably with some fluid in the urinary bladder (which we all ignored with the patient on a continuous bladder drainage). As a checklist, the continuity of the myometrium should be traced till the fundus and posteriorly to rule out rupture in every case of antepartum haemorrhage. In this case, once again it was the retracted ruptured uterus that was mistaken for a placental lobe overlying the cervix (Fig. 3.4).

This lady must have ruptured when she initially presented with bleeding to the health centre. The omental reaction and the oedematous and friable edges of the ruptured uterus put in vain all efforts to repair resulting in cut through and more bleed, and after all the struggle at repair, we decided to do a subtotal hysterectomy. The procedure and recovery were uneventful. It is therefore very important to have a high index of suspicion of rupture in every case with antepartum haemorrhage. The reason for rupture, in this case, remains unexplained.

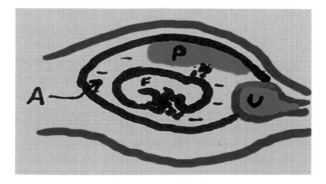

Fig. 3.4 Schematic line diagram showing the retracted uterus U mistaken as the placental lobe. The extruded foetus F is in the intact amniotic cavity with amniotic fluid A. The placenta P is anterior

3.3   Rupture Due to Misdiagnosed Malpresentation

I would like to narrate one more case which I had managed as a registrar. A woman was admitted in her third pregnancy at 37 weeks in early labour with foetal demise. She had no comorbidities. She was in spontaneous labour. She had leaked amniotic fluid from the vagina about 3 h before presenting. There was a loss of foetal movements. The admitting registrar had made a diagnosis of a breech presentation with cord prolapse with absent pulsations. The woman progressed spontaneously in labour, and when I took over the labour room, she was getting good contractions and she was fully dilated with the feet of the baby in the vagina. There was no augmentation of labour. She was not anaemic. The uterus was regularly acting. After about 1 h when she did not expel the foetus spontaneously, I decided to deliver her. The feet were in the vagina, so I gave traction to the same and uneventfully delivered the dead foetus as assisted breech delivery. It was a 2 kg foetus. What followed was a nightmare. There was postpartum haemorrhage, and when I examined the vagina, it was intact, but there was a cervical tear on the left side. It was pretty deep. I tried reaching the apex. I gave traction after suturing the highest reachable level but still could not reach the apex. I informed the consultant and arranged blood and shifted her for proceeding under general anaesthesia. In the last 1 h of struggle, her pulse had risen to 120/min and systolic BP had fallen to 90 mm of Hg. Under anaesthesia, the consultant did a vaginal exam and suspected rupture. We proceeded with laparotomy. There was rent in the lateral wall of the uterus. The stay suture taken from below was seen, and the cervical tear was continuous with the rent on the uterus. A hysterectomy was carried out. The patient recovered from the procedure well. Fortunately, there was no colporrhexis. The audit with the consultant the next day was an unforgettable experience. The notes of the admitting resident revealed that the vagina was 2 cm dilated with feet, cord, and the head tipped to the side. There were no cord pulsations. The findings clearly meant that a transverse lie had been missed. Though the labour progressed spontaneously till full dilation and the feet got delivered from the cervix into the vagina, it was truly not breech throughout labour. The lower segment must have been in impending rupture when the feet were pulled in an attempt to deliver the baby as breech. The uterus would have ruptured as the delivery was being attempted. The learning point here is that one has to be very careful while interpreting the vaginal examination findings especially when it is a compound presentation with a cord loop. I just wondered whether an intrapartum scan would have revealed that it is a transverse lie. Of course, those days (nearly 20 years back) we never had any scan facilities in the labour room. The lie may sometimes get missed because the liquor has got drained and the pelvic grip does not appear empty. I have illustrated the above case in detail though it is a known fact that labour in a transverse lie can cause rupture to bring out how subtly the detection of transverse lie can get missed especially in a labour room with high turnover and changing doctors in shift duties.

3.4   Rupture Due to Trauma of Friable Lower Segment During Caesarean Section

I faced a once in a lifetime situation about 12 years back. The registrar operating in the emergency operation theatre called me. A second gravida admitted with obstructed labour had been taken up for caesarean section. The resident had carried out lower segment caesarean section. The baby was born alive but asphyxiated. The registrar called because he could not identify the edges of the incision and had suspected extension of the lower segment incision. The baby delivery was difficult. The woman had already bled quite a lot. When I joined in, what I observed was unimaginable. The incision on the lower segment had extended all around detaching the uterus completely from the vagina at the fornix. Whereas the upper edge of the incision was seen, the lower flap was nowhere identifiable. To orient myself I had to guide a finger from the vagina below. The finger was seen from above, but the upper segment was no way connected. The cervix or lower segment was not identifiable. I had to resort to hysterectomy and closure of the vault (Fig. 3.5). It was once in a lifetime finding. The birth canal with the merged cervix and vagina must have got avulsed from the attachment to the uterocervix. It might have been in the process of impending rupture, and the caesarean incision and extraction of the baby completely disrupted the attachment of the fornix all around.

I guess the incision for the caesarean must have been low on the fused vagino-cervix (part of the birth canal in the second stage). It might be a wise idea to keep the incision in the lower segment slightly higher to avoid caesarean through colpotomy in women subjected to caesarean section late in the second stage of labour.

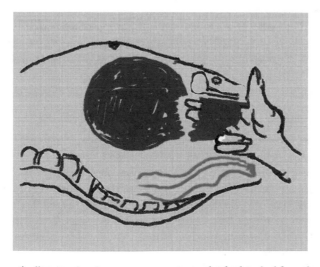

Fig. 3.5 Schematic diagram showing upper segment completely detached from the vagina

Thus, a multiparous woman would rupture when there is an obstruction to labour or when there is a transverse lie. A spontaneous rupture in the absence of these can also happen in a multiparous woman as with increasing parity few of the myometrial fibres get replaced with scar tissue. Rupture can occur in grand multiparous woman, even in the absence of labour, as has been reported by Guèye et al. [5].

In an interesting study on mice, Skurupiy and colleagues [15] observed that after repeated pregnancies the involution of myometrium gets delayed. There is hypertrophy of myometrium against poor vascularization, thereby resulting in the destruction of myocytes. The same authors [16] further confirmed that involution after third pregnancy takes longer to remove the necrosed myometrium.

3.5   Rupture of Unscarred Uterus from Literature

Rare causes of ruptured uterus in unscarred uterus have been described in the literature. Authors [14] have reported rupture of the fundus of the uterus following road traffic accident that caused foetal death and merited hysterectomy.

Sun et al. [17] reported the case of a third gravida. She had presented with upper abdominal pain at 17 weeks and later evolved into acute haemoperitoneum and shock. Laparotomy diagnosed rupture of the fundus of the uterus with intraperitoneal extrusion of the foetus. No cause could be attributed to the rupture. Various aetiologies for ruptured uterus including cocaine abuse have been reported in the literature as a cause of the uterine rupture [1]. An extremely interesting case was reported by Wang and colleagues [19]. The woman had cornual rupture but with live intact foetus in the uterus at 21 weeks. The same was managed by suturing of the rent and continuing the pregnancy. Caesarean delivery was later performed at 33 weeks of pregnancy.

Cuellar [3] reported a woman who was administered 800 μg of misoprostol for second-trimester abortion. She had previous two normal deliveries and had no scar. She developed a linear tear in the uterus which was diagnosed and sutured at laparotomy.

Syed and colleagues [18] reported a fifth gravid woman with missed abortion in the second trimester. Abortion was induced with 400 μg of misoprostol. After four doses she did not abort and so misoprostol had been repeated. She developed continuous pain. At laparotomy, she was found to have a broad ligament hematoma. On opening the same, there was a tear in the lateral wall.

In a recently published article [11], the authors observed the rate of rupture in an unscarred uterus to be 0.28 %. This study was from a large tertiary care hospital catering to women of low socioeconomic status. They observed that only 48.6 % of cases with ruptured uterus had a previous caesarean scar. 24.3 % had obstructed labour. 85.1 % had a complete rupture. Rupture involved the anterior wall in 69 %. 10.8 % had colporrhexis, and 6.8 % had associated bladder injury. A hysterectomy was necessary for 61 %. Internal iliac ligation had been performed in 2.7 % of cases. Perinatal mortality was 90.5 %, whereas maternal death occurred in 13.5 % cases. Rizwan and co-authors [12] observed similar results in their study over a 2-year period in Pakistan. They observed that prolonged neglected obstructed labour was responsible for 53.33 % of the ruptured uterus.

In a 2-year audit of ruptured uterus in a large tertiary care centre in Delhi, India, the authors [2] found that 12.6 % were in the unscarred uterus (0.04 % of the deliveries). Half of these were due to obstructed labour. Uterine malformations, administration of oxytocics, and instrumental deliveries were the other reasons for rupture in unscarred uterus.

Gibbins et al. [4] compared the ruptures in the unscarred uterus with those in the scarred uterus. They observed that the rupture in the unscarred uterus was more likely to occur in a multiparous woman and with oxytocin administration. They further observed that the maternal morbidity, hysterectomy, and perinatal mortality are significantly higher with rupture in unscarred uterus compared to rupture among women with previous caesarean section.

Thus, ruptures in an apparently unscarred uterus are usually seen in a multigravida. It can happen due to obstructed labour because of a big baby, a deflexed head with posterior position, and transverse lie in labour. Most of these ruptures would involve the lateral wall. The rupture could start in the lower segment but would invariably involve the uterine arteries. Cases with rupture due to neglected or prolonged or obstructed labour in a multiparous pregnant woman are more likely to involve the lateral wall. They are more likely to require a hysterectomy and have higher maternal mortality and perinatal deaths.

Box 3.1 summarizes the features associated with rupture of the unscarred uterus.

Box 3.1 Features of Rupture in Unscarred Uterus
Haemorrhagic shock with haemoperitoneum in labour
Loss of uterine contour and superficial foetal parts and foetal demise
Bleeding in the third or late second trimester associated with pain and loss of foetal movements
Cessation of uterine contractions in labour with or without bleeding from the vagina
Profound foetal bradycardia invariably resulting in foetal demise in labour
Recession of presenting part
Inability to feel foetal parts through the cervix
Brisk postpartum haemorrhage
Intrapartum or postpartum haematuria

References

1. Agarwal R, Gupta B, Radhakrishnan G. Rupture of the intrapartum unscarred uterus at the fundus: a complication of passive cocaine abuse? Arch Gynecol Obstet. 2011;283 Suppl 1:53–4. doi:10.1007/s00404-011-1853-6. Epub 2011 Feb 17.

2. Batra K, Gaikwad HS, Gutgutia I, Prateek S, Bajaj B. Determinants of rupture of the unscarred uterus and the related feto-maternal outcome: a current scenario in a low-income country. Trop Doct. 2016;46(2):69–73. doi:10.1177/0049475515598464. Epub 2015 Aug 13.
3. Cuellar Torriente M. Silent uterine rupture with the use of misoprostol for second-trimester termination of pregnancy: a case report. Obstet Gynecol Int. 2011;2011:584652. doi:10.1155/2011/584652. Epub 2011 Apr 19.
4. Gibbins KJ, Weber T, Holmgren CM, Porter TF, Varner MW, Manuck TA. Maternal and fetal morbidity associated with uterine rupture of the unscarred uterus. Am J Obstet Gynecol. 2015;213(3):382. doi:10.1016/j.ajog.2015.05.048.e1-6. Epub 2015 May 28.
5. Guèye M, Mbaye M, Ndiaye-Guèye MD, Kane-Guèye SM, Diouf AA, Niang MM, Diaw H, Moreau JC. Spontaneous uterine rupture of an unscarred uterus before labour. Case Rep Obstet Gynecol. 2012;2012:598356. doi:10.1155/2012/598356. Epub 2012 Dec 3.
6. Guiliano M, Closset E, Therby D, LeGoueff F, Deruelle P, Subtil D. Signs, symptoms and complications of complete and partial uterine ruptures during pregnancy and delivery. Eur J Obstet Gynecol Reprod Biol. 2014;179:130–4 (ISSN: 1872-7654).
7. Gupta A, Nanda S. Uterine rupture in pregnancy: a five-year study. Arch Gynecol Obstet. 2011;283(3):437–41. doi:10.1007/s00404-010-1357-9. Epub 2010 Jan 28.
8. Khooharo Y, Yousfani JZ, Malik SH, Amber A, Majeed N, Malik NH, Pervez H, Majeed I, Majeed N. Incidence and management of rupture uterus in obstructed labour. J Ayub Med Coll Abbottabad. 2013;25(1–2):149–51.
9. Matsuo K, Scanlon JT, Atlas RO, Kopelman JN. Staircase sign: a newly described uterine contraction pattern seen in rupture of the unscarred gravid uterus. J Obstet Gynaecol Res. 2008;34(1):100–4 (ISSN: 1341-8076).
10. Prajapati P, Sheikh MI, Patel R. Case report rupture uterus: carelessness or negligence? J Indian Acad Forensic Med. 2012;34(1):82. ISSN 0971-0973.
11. Rathod S, Samal SK, Swain S. A three year clinicopathological study of cases of rupture uterus. J Clin Diagn Res. 2015;9(11):QC04–6. doi:10.7860/JCDR/2015/14554.6783. Epub 2015 Nov 1.
12. Rizwan N, Abbasi RM, Uddin SF. Uterine rupture, the frequency of cases and fetomaternal outcome. J Pak Med Assoc. 2011;61(4):322–4.
13. Singh A, Shrivastava C. Uterine rupture: still a harsh reality! J Obstet Gynaecol India. 2015;65(3):158–61. doi:10.1007/s13224-014-0551-2. Epub 2014 Jul 5.
14. Sisay Woldeyes W, Amenu D, Segni H. Uterine rupture in pregnancy following fall from a motorcycle: a horrid accident in pregnancy-a case report and review of the literature. Case Rep Obstet Gynecol. 2015;2015:715180. doi:10.1155/2015/715180. Epub 2015 Oct 21.
15. Skurupiy VA, Obedinskaya KS, Nadeev AP. Structural manifestations of mechanisms of myometrium involution after repeated pregnancies in mice. Bull Exp Biol Med. 2010;149(5):554–8.
16. Skurupiy VA, Obedinskaya KS, Nadeev AP. Morphological study of the main mechanisms of myometrium involution after repeated pregnancies in mice. Bull Exp Biol Med. 2011;150(3):378–82.
17. Sun HD, Su WH, Chang WH, Wen L, Huang BS, Wang PH. Rupture of a pregnant unscarred uterus in an early secondary trimester: a case report and brief review. J Obstet Gynaecol Res. 2012;38(2):442–5. doi:10.1111/j.1447-0756.2011.01723.x. Epub 2012 Jan 10.
18. Syed S, Noreen H, Kahloon LE, Chaudhri R. Uterine rupture associated with the use of intravaginal misoprostol during second-trimester pregnancy termination. J Pak Med Assoc. 2011;61(4):399–401.
19. Wang PH, Chao HT, Too LL, Yuan CC. Primary repair of cornual rupture occurring at 21 weeks gestation and successful pregnancy outcome. Hum Reprod. 1999;14(7):1894–5.
20. Xia X, Fan L, Xia Y, Fang Y. Uterine rupture during pregnancy. Clin Exp Obstet Gynecol. 2011;38(3):286–7.

Rupture of the Uterus Weakened Due to Rare Causes

4

The search for newer and newer conservative approach for averting hysterectomy in a patient with atonic PPH has had its journey till B-lynch suture established itself as an accepted standard technique [3].

4.1   Rupture Due to Previous Compression Sutures

I would like to narrate the following case. A woman pregnant for the second time presented at 24 weeks of pregnancy with shock. She had no live children. She experienced severe abdominal pain and bleeding from the vagina 1 h before the presentation. On examination, she was in haemorrhagic shock with obvious features of haemoperitoneum and superficial foetal parts and absent foetal heart sounds. At laparotomy, there was more than a litre of haemoperitoneum. It was agonizing to find a Z-shaped ragged rupture of the anterior wall of the upper segment (Fig. 4.1a). The dead foetus was lying in the peritoneal cavity. The edges were briskly bleeding. I had to resort to hysterectomy. The procedure and recovery were uneventful. The past obstetric history available in her documents was a wake-up call. The woman had been admitted in her first pregnancy to our hospital with a diagnosis of abruption and foetal demise due to preeclampsia at term. Labour had been induced, and she delivered. There was a massive atonic postpartum haemorrhage. Systematic devascularization and internal iliac artery ligation failed to arrest bleeding. In a desperate attempt to save the uterus, as she was nulliparous, the consultant had given box sutures in the anterior wall of the uterus (Fig. 4.1b) to compress it tightly. The sutures succeeded in controlling the bleeding, and the uterus was conserved. She had an uneventful recovery after receiving multiple blood and component transfusions.

It was the bites of the box suture in the upper segment given at the previous laparotomy that behaved like an upper segment scar and ruptured in the second trimester of the subsequent pregnancy. It is therefore very important to understand that no compression sutures should ever involve taking bites through the upper segment of the uterus.

© Springer Nature Singapore Pte Ltd. 2017
G. Dorairajan, *Ruptured Uterus*, DOI 10.1007/978-981-10-2852-6_4

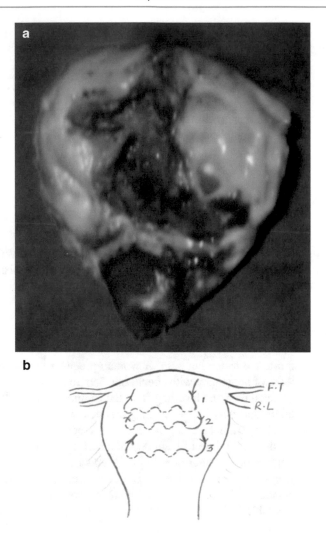

Fig. 4.1 (**a**) A photograph of the hysterectomy specimen showing Z-shaped tear in the upper seg-ment. (**b**) Schematic diagram of the box compression sutures (*1,2,3*) applied in the upper segment. *F.T* fallopian tube and *R.L* round ligament (Reproduced with permission from *J Obstet Gynecol* India. Vol 57, No. 1: January/February 2006, Page 79–80)

4.2   Rupture After Previous Manual Removal of Placenta

It is mysterious how and when the upper segment becomes weak.

I encountered this case about 14 years back. A woman presented in her second pregnancy at 36 weeks of gestation with breech presentation and premature rupture of membranes. The index pregnancy was spontaneous conception. In the first pregnancy 2 years back, she had a spontaneous vaginal delivery attended at home by an untrained attendant. There was a history of difficult placental delivery. She had presented to our hospital 3 days after delivery with features of grade IV puerperal sepsis with frank peritonitis. A laparotomy then revealed 1 l of pus in the peritoneal cavity with a puerperal uterus. Peritoneal lavage and drainage were carried out. She had made an uneventful recovery and had been discharged after 10 days of hospital stay. Given premature rupture of membranes with flexed breech presentation, caesarean section was decided and performed. To our immense surprise, there was a ragged old rent in the fundus of the uterus through which the membranes were bulging out. A lower segment incision delivered a 2.2 kg baby. The edge of the fundal rent was freshened for repair, but the wide ragged edges with bleeding compelled me to perform a hysterectomy (Fig. 4.2). I could only thank the Almighty for giving her breech presentation without labour and thus making our decision for caesarean clear cut. If only she had gone into spontaneous or induced labour, there would have been a calamity. Some women are indeed lucky.

Manual removal of the placenta has been associated with problems. A forceful removal of an adherent placental lobe could result in weakening resulting in bleeding infection or even rupture.

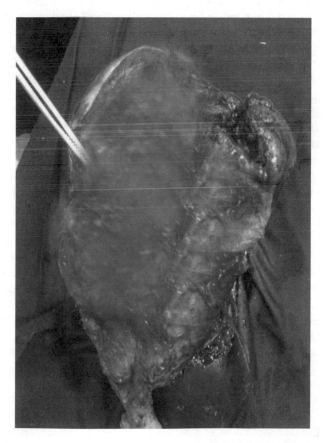

Fig. 4.2 The hysterectomy specimen showing ragged rent in the fundus of the uterus

Akinola et al. [2] reported a multiparous woman whose third stage was attended by an untrained attendant. There was difficulty in removal of placenta which was attempted by the attendant. She developed a rupture of the uterus with the evisceration of the bowel through the uterine rent protruding from the vagina. It is rare to see such incidents.

Zwart and colleagues [7] reported the second gravida with life-threatening bleeding due to ruptured uterus that occurred while doing a manual removal of the retained placenta. She required hysterectomy and embolization. She had earlier undergone curettage for abortion. Thus retained placenta is also a feature of abnormal placentation and a preexisting possible weakness in the myometrium that could form a rent when attempting forceful manual removal of the placenta.

4.3   Rupture of Uterus Weakened Due to Previous Intrauterine Procedures

The weakening of the uterus could be brought about by curettage or perforation or any intrauterine procedure where the complication remains silent and weakens the uterus. It comes to light only after a mishap like a rupture or adherent placenta in the subsequent pregnancy. Something similar happened in the following case.

The patient was a known case of rheumatic heart disease NYHA II. She had an uneventful caesarean section for foetal distress 4 years back. She presented with premature rupture of membranes at 26 weeks of pregnancy. She was kept on conservative management awaiting spontaneous onset of labour. We counselled her about the risks of infection in the wake of underlying rheumatic heart disease. All the liquor had drained. After 1 week she developed mild unexplained tachycardia. Suspecting the onset of an infection, the woman and her husband were counselled again, and decision for termination was taken. Labour was induced with misoprostol tablet 200 mg orally as the fundal height was just 24 weeks size. After the second dose, she went into labour. But another 3 h later, she complained of severe pain and was in shock. I felt miserable for the decision of misoprostol for induction and suspected scar rupture. Urgent laparotomy was carried out. We presumed that the lower caesarean scar had ruptured. At laparotomy, there was 700 ml haemoperitoneum. The foetus had been extruded into the peritoneal cavity from a 5 cm rent in the fundus of the uterus (Fig. 4.3a) with the placenta still in the uterus. The lower segment which confirmed features suggestive of previous lower segment caesarean scar was intact. The rent was successfully repaired (Fig. 4.3b) and bilateral tubectomy carried out after informed consent. On further questioning in the postoperative period, the only significant history was of an intrauterine copper contraceptive device inserted 6 weeks after the last delivery in a local health centre that had been removed 6 months before the present pregnancy. Since the documents of the previous surgery had confirmed it to be an uneventful lower segment caesarean, I presume the weakening of the upper segment might be due to IUCD which might have burrowed deeper than the mucosa or a small perforation sustained during insertion.

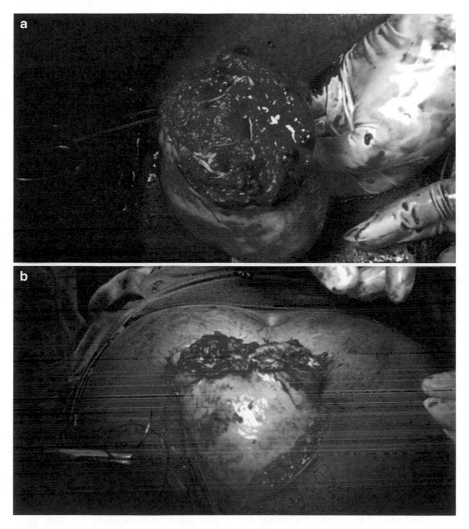

Fig. 4.3 (a) A large rent on the fundus of the uterus through which the foetus was extruded. (b) The rent has been sutured

A similar case was reported by Smid and co-authors [6] in a 42-year-old woman with twin to twin transfusion syndrome who had a rupture of the posterior wall in her pregnancy. It was presumably due to an unrecognized scar of a displaced IUCD. Juong and colleagues [4] reported a case that had one-term caesarean and a dilation and curettage for a missed abortion earlier. She was confirmed to have choriodecidual separation and fever at 21 weeks of pregnancy. Caesarean done at 27 weeks for foetal distress revealed a fundal rupture at a site probably weakened by the previous curettage. The chorioamniotic separation had also started at the same site.

Abdalla and colleagues [1] reported a woman at 28 weeks of pregnancy with progressively increasing pain in the lower abdomen. She was taken for laparotomy given suspected haemoperitoneum. A large 10 cm rent was seen in the posterior wall. This woman previously had a normal delivery and curettage for a miscarriage. There was no history suggestive of perforation during the curettage. The uterus must have become weakened in the posterior wall following the procedure. There was no other possible cause of rupture identified in their case.

Nishijima et al. [5] reported rupture of the uterus in a subsequent pregnancy at 26 weeks in a woman who had earlier undergone resection of the interstitial portion of the fallopian tube for an interstitial ectopic pregnancy.

Thus, rupture can also occur in women whose uterus has become weak at some place due to previous procedures like curettage, manual removal of placenta, etc. It is very difficult to anticipate or predict as to which case could have a problem. It is therefore not wise to advocate an elective caesarean for all these cases. The uterus could rupture in labour or silently as the uterus distends. It can also happen when pregnancy is terminated in the second trimester for some reason. Most of these are retrospective revelations. Most of these ruptures would involve the upper segment as a ragged rent requiring a hysterectomy. They are also associated with high perinatal mortality and maternal morbidity.

References

1. Abdalla N, Reinholz-Jaskolska M, Bachanek M, Cendrowski K, Stanczak R, Sawicki W. Hemoperitoneum in a patient with spontaneous rupture of the posterior wall of an unscarred uterus in the second trimester of pregnancy. BMC Res Notes. 2015;8:603. doi:10.1186/s13104-015-1575-0. Published online 2015 Oct 24.
2. Akinola OI, Fabamwo AO, Oludara B, Akinola RA, Oshodi YA, Adebayo SK. Ruptured uterus and bowel injury from manual removal of placenta: a case report. Niger Postgrad Med J. 2012;19(3):181–3.
3. B-Lynch C, Coker A, Lawal AH, et al. The B-Lynch surgical technique for the control of massive postpartum haemorrhage: an alternative to hysterectomy? Five cases reported. Br J Obstet Gynaecol. 1997;104:372–5.
4. Joung EJ, You SK, Lee JY, Ahn JW, Yun NR, Hwang SO. A live birth after spontaneous complete chorioamniotic membrane separation associated with a uterine scar. Obstet Gynecol Sci. 2016;59(2):144–7. doi:10.5468/ogs.2016.59.2.144. Epub 2016 Mar 16.
5. Nishijima Y, Suzuki T, Kashiwagi H, Narita A, Kanno H, Hayashi M, Shinoda M, Noji C, Mitsuzuka K, Nishimura O, Ishimoto H. Uterine rupture at 26 weeks of pregnancy following laparoscopic salpingectomy with resection of the interstitial portion: a case report. Tokai J Exp Clin Med. 2014;39(4):169–71 (ISSN: 2185–2243).
6. Smid MC, Waltner-Toews R, Goodnight W. Spontaneous posterior uterine rupture in twin-twin transfusion syndrome. AJP Rep. 2016;6(1):e68–70. doi:10.1055/s-0035-1566243. Epub 2015 Nov 16.
7. Zwart JJ, van Huisseling HC, Schuttevaer HM, van Roosmalen J, Oepkes D. Nearly fatal uterine rupture during manual removal of the placenta: a case report. J Reprod Med. 2007;52(10):974–6.

Rupture in a Primigravida

5

5.1   Rupture Following Obstructed Labour

The traditional teaching is that multigravidae rupture their uterus and primigravidae go for secondary inertia or arrest of labour or exhaustion. I would like to narrate a case I had seen 20 years back in the emergency room. A primigravida was brought to the emergency room by her husband and mother. Her husband had lifted her on his shoulders. Their journey to the hospital had taken 2 days changing from bullock carts to buses from a nearby state. When the husband seated the woman on the bench, the woman had the look of death on her face. She could barely move. The face was expressionless. It had surpassed all the possible pain. The eyes were sunken. She was severely pale. She had not eaten anything for 2 days and was in labour for more than a day before undertaking this journey. She had tachycardia. The blood pressure was 90/60 mm of Hg. Abdomen revealed tenderness all over with distension and absent foetal heart sounds. She was febrile. Vaginal examination revealed pus and slough at the vault. Cervix could not be delineated. The head was high up. I have never since encountered a case with such findings on vaginal examination. After resuscitation laparotomy was carried out. Laparotomy revealed a sloughed off lower segment. The head was visible through it. The lower edge of the lower segment was friable and oedematous. The sigmoid colon and bladder appeared unhealthy oedematous and blue. The foetus was extracted out. Hysterectomy was carried out. Prolonged continued bladder drainage failed to prevent vesicovaginal fistula. Eventually, she developed a high rectal fistula. Vaginal examination 2 weeks later revealed only sloughed out tissue everywhere in the pelvis with faeces and urine pouring from the vagina. Such agonizing could be the misery of obstructed labour. How cruel the health system could be which fails to prevent such a misery that even death would look like a gift. Fortunately, we can take pride that the whole health system has improved drastically with the upgrading of primary centres and community health centres to provide emergency obstetric services. In this case, the rupture was probably due to pressure necrosis and sloughing off of the lower segment due to prolonged pressure necrosis and infection as the

© Springer Nature Singapore Pte Ltd. 2017
G. Dorairajan, *Ruptured Uterus*, DOI 10.1007/978-981-10-2852-6_5

patient was probably in active labour for nearly 36–48 h. Fortunate are the present-day residents who would never see such situations.

Chigbu and colleagues [4] reported ruptured uterus in a primigravida due to obstructed labour. The woman reported was 40 years old and was in obstructed labour. She had a rupture of the anterior lower segment with a stillbirth. There was no history of any previous uterine procedure.

It is very rare to find a primigravida with obstructed labour going in for rupture as the uterus goes in for secondary inertia. It can happen when oxytocics are used to augment labour in them to overcome the secondary inertia not realizing that there is obstructed labour due to either malposition or cephalopelvic disproportion.

5.2   Rupture of the Posterior Wall

I would like to narrate the following case just to bring out that the birth attendant who persists and tries to deliver with undue fundal pressure failing to recognize obstructed labour can do a lot of harm.

A primigravida was referred from a health centre late in labour.

She had been in labour for nearly 16 h before she presented. At admission, she was exhausted and dehydrated and had tachycardia. The blood pressure was normal. The abdomen revealed features of obstructed labour with a big baby. The foetal heart rate was 110/min. There was secondary inertia. Vaginal examination revealed vertex at 0 station with a large caput reaching till introitus and irreversible mould-ing. There was thick meconium stained liquor. An emergency caesarean section was performed. The peritoneal fluid was blood stained (200 ml). The lower segment was stretched. The caesarean section was uneventful. An asphyxiated foetus weighing 3.5 kg was born. The uterine incision was sutured. On examining the posterior sur-face of the uterus near the fundus, we observed 3 cm area of a bruise with slow ooze (Fig. 5.1). The same was sutured.

The woman later confirmed the use of continued fundal pressure by the birth attendant in an overenthusiastic effort to deliver the patient. I have never imagined such a possible fate after fundal pressure. It was an eye opener. Fundal pressure should be discouraged by all means. Rupture of the posterior wall in the absence of previous surgery like myomectomy, etc. is extremely rare. Rupture invariably occurs in the anterior wall being the thinnest or in lateral wall in a multigravida with neglected labour. Abdalla and colleagues [1] reported a woman with increasing pain and features of free fluid and falling haemoglobin at 28 weeks of pregnancy. The foetus was doing well. Laparotomy revealed a posterior wall rent with 1 l of haemo-peritoneum. They could not identify any cause.

Matsubara and co-authors [6] reported an interesting case. A 27-year-old primi-gravida had presented at term with irregular uterine contractions. A hard mass was felt anteriorly which was diagnosed to be thinned out bulging anterior uterine wall with foetal parts in it. An incomplete rupture was confirmed by caesarean section. Long-standing sacculation of the uterus was proposed to be the reason for thinning and incomplete rupture.

Fig. 5.1 Photograph showing disruption due to bruising at the fundus of the uterus

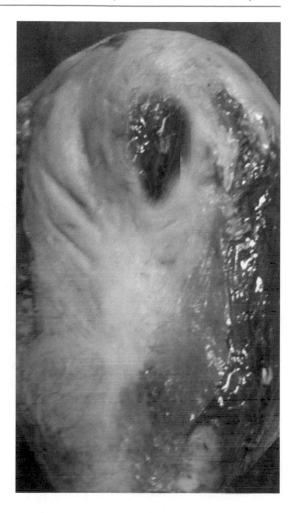

Rupture of the mid posterior wall of the uterus was reported by Takeda et al. [12] in a primigravida at 32 weeks of pregnancy. She had undergone uterine artery embolization for a cervical ectopic pregnancy 4 years earlier. A similar case of rupture was reported [13] in a woman pregnant after uterine artery embolization for fibroid uterus. She was also found to have abnormal placentation in the form of placenta percreta invading through the layers at the site of rupture.

5.3   Iatrogenic Extraperitoneal Disruption of Uterine Artery Due to Instrumental Delivery

I would like to narrate one more case with iatrogenic cause. The second gravida with previous normal delivery was admitted in labour. The pregnancy was otherwise uncomplicated. There were no comorbidities. The labour progressed well, but in the second stage, the descent of the head was a little delayed. It was slightly mal-rotated head at +2 station. The estimated weight was 3.2 kg. There were no features of cephalopelvic disproportion. In an enthusiastic attempt to deliver, the registrar had applied low forceps. It was a difficult delivery. The baby was born alive but had low Apgar score at birth. There was a deep tear in the left lateral vaginal wall. There was a linear tear in the cervix on the left side. The registrar had sutured the same. The patient did not require any blood transfusion. Two days after delivery, she appeared pale. The pulse was a 100 per minute. The blood pressure was normal. Examination of the abdomen revealed a large oblique mass on the left side from above pubic symphysis occupying the left iliac fossa. Vaginal examination and scan confirmed it to be a left broad ligament hematoma.

Since she was stable, the woman was managed conservatively. Broad-spectrum antibiotics were administered, and two bottles of blood were transfused. There was no further drop in the haemoglobin. There was no pyrexia. After 10 days the hematoma size started shrinking becoming firmer, and after 3 months, it got completely absorbed. Though truly this is not a ruptured uterus, I have described the case because it is rupture of the uterine artery on the left side probably due to the direct extension of the cervical tear. It is possible that the apex was not visualized properly at the time of the primary suturing of the tear. The woman was lucky that the hematoma contained itself to the broad ligament and was self-limiting because of the tamponade effect. However, it is a matter of great concern as it added to the morbidity and the need for the transfusions, and it also extended the hospital stay. Unfortunately, we don't have her follow-up of subsequent pregnancies as it is a matter of worry that she might rupture her uterus during labour in the subsequent pregnancy.

5.4   Rupture Following Induction of Labour

It is indeed rare for a primigravida to rupture her uterus. Most often there is an iatrogenic element including the injudicious use of oxytocics. The following case is just to bring out how communication gaps can prove dangerous.

A primigravida was admitted at 41 weeks of pregnancy. On examination she was normotensive. She was not anaemic. There were no comorbidities. Abdomen revealed single foetus in right occipito-anterior position with adequate liquor, good foetal heart sounds, and an estimated weight of 3 kg. Ultrasonography confirmed the same. The pelvis was normal. The Bishop score was 4. We planned induction of labour. The cervix was ripened with prostaglandin E2 gel. After 12 h the Bishop score was favourable. 25 micrograms of misoprostol were administered vaginally 4th hourly. After two doses she was in established active labour. Membranes were ruptured artificially at 5 cm dilation. The liquor was clear. The vertex had descended to -1 station. After about 3 h she complained of severe sudden pain lower abdomen and shoulder tip pain. The pulse had risen to 120/min, and blood pressure was 90 systolic. The uterine contractions had ceased. The abdomen was diffusely tender, and the foetal heart sounds were no longer heard. There was bleeding from vagina noted. Suspecting rupture she was taken for urgent laparotomy. There was rupture of the lower segment, and the foetus was in the abdominal cavity. There was 1 l of haemoperitoneum. The foetus was extracted and the lower segment was repaired. On critically analysing the case, it was observed that the third dose of misoprostol had been administered by the staff nurse within half hour of the artificial rupture of membranes because the dose was due. It is very important to understand and delay the administration of the due dose of prostaglandins if the contractions are moderate and artificial rupture of membranes (ARM) has been done because ARM would further augment the contractions. It was very tragic and a wake-up call for the whole team. The labour had got further enhanced after rupturing of membranes and not realizing the third dose of misoprostol had been administered by the staff nurse as there were no written instructions not to do so. In service hospital where the doctor-patient ratio is poor and the nurses are carrying out the administration of drugs, the instructions should be spelled out clearly. Any communication gap between the doctors/residents and the other members of the team administering drugs could prove very costly to patient care. After this incidence we developed safety strategies and protocols for administering inducing agents.

Chen et al. recently published a systematic review [2]. The authors concluded that vaginal misoprostol was very effective in achieving delivery within 24 h but was found to have a high risk of hyperstimulation and foetal compromise compared to oral misoprostol or mechanical method of induction.

Thus, one has to be very careful while using prostaglandins for induction of labour even in a primigravida.

Mourad and colleagues [9] reported a 23-year-old woman who ruptured her uterus after premature rupture of membranes at 32 weeks of pregnancy even before she went in for established labour. There was no induction of labour. They could not establish a cause. Mishina and colleagues [7] reported another interesting case. They diagnosed a large defect in the fundus of the uterus of a primigravida at 32 weeks of gestation who complained of severe abdominal pain. The cause for the weakening of the myometrium could not be established.

5.5 Rupture Due to Uterine Malformations

Malformations of the uterus have been found to increase the risk of rupture. The condition can be diagnosed early in symptomatic women with imaging. We came across a primigravida at 10 weeks of pregnancy with abdominal pain. She had continuous moderate pain on the right side. She was otherwise stable. Sonography made us suspect a rudimentary horn pregnancy. Laparotomy revealed unruptured cornual pregnancy of a rudimentary horn. The noncommunicating horn with pregnancy was excised (Fig. 5.2).

If missed in early pregnancy, the horn may eventually rupture as happened in the following case. A primigravida presented at 16 weeks of amenorrhoea with features of haemorrhagic shock. There was haemoperitoneum and diffuse tenderness in the abdomen. Laparotomy confirmed a ruptured cornual pregnancy. Cornual resection

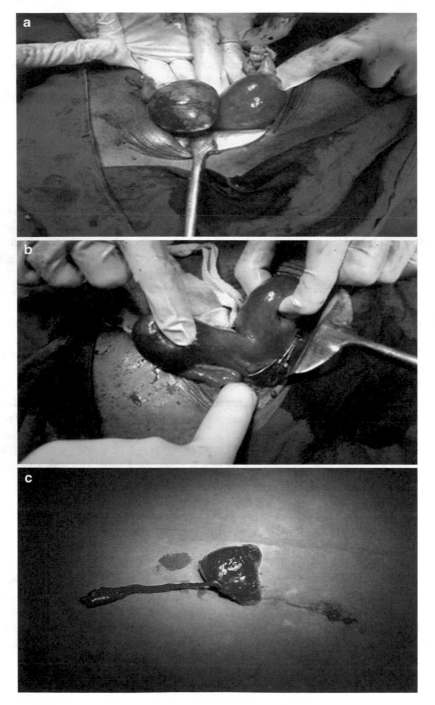

Fig. 5.2 (a) Unruptured cornual pregnancy. (b) The rudimentary horn was a noncommunicating type. (c) The same was excised

was done. Interstitial ectopic pregnancy is a close differential diagnosis in a woman presenting around 14–16 weeks with shock and haemoperitoneum. Spontaneous rupture of cornual or interstitial pregnancies would typically occur around 14–16 weeks of pregnancy. The location of the round ligament helps in differentiating between the two entities. The round ligament would be medial to the rupture site in interstitial pregnancies. There are umpteen cases reported in the literature of rupture of cornual pregnancy. Diagnosis before rupture is possible with MRI, and management with minimally invasive surgery has been reported [5, 11].

Mizutamari and colleagues [8] reported yet another interesting case of a defect in the fundus near the cornual region of a primigravida with an unscarred uterus at 32 weeks. The woman was asymptomatic. Imaging diagnosed a defect with bulging amniotic membrane. Emergency caesarean section was performed. There was perforation near right cornual region. Follow-up hysterography diagnosed an arcuate uterus. The focal thinning of myometrium in the cornual region was proposed to be due to Mullerian abnormality.

Chen and colleagues [3] reported an unusual case of a primigravida. The woman was a known case of endometriosis and had presented with excessive intermenstrual bleed. She was found to have a ruptured endometrioma of the posterior cervicovaginal junction that had ruptured and was bleeding. The same was evacuated and repaired. In the subsequent pregnancy during labour, she had a rupture of this posterior cervical wound that extended to the lateral wall of the lower segment. In the case reported by Nikolaou et al. [10], a 33-year-old primigravida was suspected to have ruptured uterus at 28 weeks of pregnancy on the basis of abnormal foetal heart rate pattern and haemoperitoneum. Laparotomy revealed a large fundal rupture. Histopathology of the hysterectomy specimen had confirmed an adenomyosis.

Thus, a primigravida could rupture her uterus when there is a malformation of the uterus with pregnancy in the noncommunicating rudimentary horn. It is extremely rare to develop rupture after obstructed labour. Injudicious use of labour-inducing agents poses a risk of hyperstimulation and could result in rupture. Most of the ruptures in the primigravida are associated with poor perinatal outcome.

References

1. Abdalla N, Reinholz-Jaskolska M, Bachanek M, Cendrowski K, Stanczak R, Sawicki W. Hemoperitoneum in a patient with spontaneous rupture of the posterior wall of an unscarred uterus in the second trimester of pregnancy. BMC Res Notes. 2015;8:603. doi:10.1186/s13104-015-1575-0. Published online 2015 Oct 24.
2. Chen W, Xue J, Peprah MK, Wen SW, Walker M, Gao Y, Tang YA. Systematic review and network meta-analysis comparing the use of Foley catheters, misoprostol, and dinoprostone for cervical ripening in the induction of labour. BJOG. 2016;123(3):346–54. doi:10.1111/1471-0528.13456. Epub 2015 Nov 5.
3. Chen ZH, Chen M, Tsai HD, Wu CH. Intrapartum uterine rupture associated with a scarred cervix because of a previous rupture of cystic cervical endometriosis. Taiwan J Obstet Gynecol. 2011;50(1):95–7. doi:10.1016/j.tjog.2009.05.001.
4. Chigbu B, Onwere S, Kamanu C, Aluka C, Adibe E, Onichakwe C. Rupture of the uterus in a primigravida: a case report. Niger J Clin Pract. 2010;13(2):233–4.

5. Lennox G, Pantazi S, Keunen J, Van Mieghem T, Allen L. Minimally invasive surgical management of a second-trimester pregnancy in a rudimentary uterine horn. J Obstet Gynaecol Can. 2013;35(5):468–72.
6. Matsubara S, Shimada K, Kuwata T, Usui R, Suzuki M. Thin anterior uterine wall with incomplete uterine rupture in a primigravida detected by palpation and ultrasound: a case report. J Med Case Rep. 2011;5:14. doi:10.1186/1752-1947-5-14.
7. Mishina M, Hasegawa J, Ichizuka K, Oba T, Sekizawa A, Okai T. Defect in the uterine wall with prolapse of amniotic sac into it at 32 weeks' gestation in a primigravida woman without any previous uterine surgery. J Obstet Gynaecol Res. 2014;40(3):840–2. doi:10.1111/jog.12214. Epub 2013 Nov 18.
8. Mizutamari E, Honda T, Ohba T, Katabuchi H. Spontaneous rupture of an unscarred gravid uterus in a primigravid woman at 32 weeks of gestation. Case Rep Obstet Gynecol. 2014;2014:209585. doi:10.1155/2014/209585. Published online 2014 Jun 30.
9. Mourad WS, Bersano DJ, Greenspan PB, Harper DM. Spontaneous rupture of the unscarred uterus in a primigravida with preterm prelabour rupture of membranes. BMJ Case Rep. 2015;2015:pii: bcr2014207321. doi:10.1136/bcr-2014-207321.
10. Nikolaou M, Kourea HP, Antonopoulos K, Geronatsiou K, Adonakis G, Decavalas G. Spontaneous uterine rupture in a primigravida woman in the early third trimester attributed to adenomyosis: a case report and review of the literature. J Obstet Gynaecol Res. 2013;39(3):727–32 (ISSN: 1447-0756).
11. Singh P, Gupta R, Das B, Bajaj SK, Misra R. Midtrimester spontaneous torsion of unruptured gravid rudimentary horn: presurgical diagnosis on magnetic resonance imaging. J Obstet Gynaecol Res. 2015;41(9):1478–82. doi:10.1111/jog.12722. Epub 2015 May 27.
12. Takeda J, Makino S, Ota A, Tawada T, Mitsuhashi N, Takeda S. Spontaneous uterine rupture at 32 weeks of gestation after previous uterine artery embolization. J Obstet Gynaecol Res. 2014;40(1):243–6 (ISSN: 1447-0756).
13. Yeaton-Massey A, Loring M, Chetty S, Druzin M. Uterine rupture after uterine artery embolization for symptomatic leiomyomas. Obstet Gynecol. 2014;123(2 Pt 2 Suppl 2):418–20 (ISSN: 1873-233X).

Rupture of The Uterus Weakened by Myomectomy Scars

6

6.1   Rupture Following Open Resection of Myoma

Fibroid uterus is a known cause of infertility as well as recurrent preterm losses. Myomectomy in selected cases improves the pregnancy rates as well as outcomes. However, there is an increased risk of rupture in subsequent pregnancy at term or in labour, more so in cases where the cavity had been entered or where extensive myometrial tunnelling had been done. So these pregnancies are well-anticipated volcanoes. I can never forget this case I encountered about 18 years back. A third gravid woman was admitted to our hospital. She had previous two preterm deliveries; both the babies had died in the neonatal intensive care unit due to extreme prematurity. She was found to have a large fibroid for which she had undergone myomectomy, before conceiving the third time. The documentation was unequivocal. A large anterior wall intramural myoma had been removed. The uterine cavity had been opened. She was under close supervision from the beginning of this pregnancy. We admitted her at 28 weeks of pregnancy. We planned an elective caesarean section for her at 34 weeks of pregnancy (end of the same week of the fateful day). There were no antenatal complications. The foetus was growing well. All investigations were normal. Anaesthetists had been consulted, and blood availability had been ensured. Elective caesarean section was scheduled in 2 days time. On a fateful night, she complained of shoulder tip pain and epigastric pain. The blood pressure was normal. There was mild tachycardia. Before one could recognize and realize, the abdominal examination revealed foetal bradycardia. She was in the operation theatre within 10 min, but alas it had become a full-blown rupture. The foetus had been extruded into the abdominal cavity, and there was large rent in the upper segment. She lost not only the baby but also her uterus. She had an otherwise uneventful recovery. I still remember clearly the bed on which she had stayed all this while. It was indeed very agonizing. It makes me wonder why God is so cruel to a few. Why a few women come very close but never get to mother a child? It leaves me wondering about the mysterious, powerful universal force that operates and limits human endeavour.

© Springer Nature Singapore Pte Ltd. 2017   51
G. Dorairajan, *Ruptured Uterus*, DOI 10.1007/978-981-10-2852-6_6

Lenihan and colleagues [5] reported a case where shoulder tip pain was the only symptom alerting about a likely rupture in a patient who was under epidural analgesia during labour.

6.2   Rupture Following Previous Laparoscopic Myomectomy

Advances in science and technology with easy accessibility, affordability, and availability of artificial reproductive technology and minimally invasive surgery have proven to be a boon to a few helping them enjoy motherhood. However, at the same time, it has added to a whole new list of morbidity and mortality due to problems of abnormal placentation and higher age group-related medical problems. I would like to narrate the following case I recently encountered; another case as a testimony to the mystery of the powerful universal force. A 38-year-old woman had conceived with in vitro fertilization procedure. She had been infertile and undergone treatment for many years. She had been diagnosed with endometriosis and myoma uterus. Laparoscopic myomectomy of an anterior wall fibroid along with adhesiolysis was performed on her 2 years prior. She presented at 28 weeks of pregnancy with pain abdomen to our hospital. There was no bleeding from the vagina. She was not hypertensive. It was a singleton pregnancy. The resident duty team and the junior consultant had seen and managed the case. At admission the pulse was 110/min. Blood pressure was 120/70 mm of Hg. The patient was pale. Her BMI was 35. Morbid obesity obscured the abdominal findings. Contour was well made out, and foetal heart was difficult to localize clinically. Foetal heart activity was localized and confirmed to be normal on sonography. The uterus was not tense. We transfused two bottles of whole blood as she was severely anaemic. After 4 h suddenly the patient collapsed, with the low volume pulse of 120/min and blood pressure not recordable. She was severely pale. Abdominal examination revealed diffuse tenderness. Bedside ultrasound examination confirmed foetal demise and intrauterine death and free fluid in the peritoneal cavity. Even before the patient was wheeled in for laparotomy, she arrested and died. Such a drastic happening is an agony. On critically analysing the case, I realized there must have been concealed abruption to start with, which explains the pain and pallor but a live foetus at admission. The rising intrauterine tension must have resulted in rupture through the myometrium weakened due to laparoscopic myomectomy. The resulting rupture must have resulted in sudden brisk exsanguination in an already pale and compromised patient. It is very important to have a high index of suspicion of abruption in unexplained pain and pallor in the presence of a live foetus. A high index of suspicion is also needed for rupture in cases with laparoscopic myomectomy even though the documents may confirm that the cavity has not been opened. Whether this case started rupturing right at admission is contentious because the foetus was alive. Usually, rupture occurs near term or in labour in a woman who have had a myomectomy. Rupture can get initiated earlier even before she is in labour if the intrauterine tension is high. Multiple pregnancies, polyhydramnios, and concealed haemorrhage as possibly, in this case, can increase the intrauterine tension. The increased intrauterine pressure can result in rupture of the uterus at the site of weakened myomectomy scar.

6.3 Literature Review of Rupture After Myomectomy and Discussion

Many authors have reported a rupture in the third trimester after laparoscopic myomectomy [3, 9, 11]. Matsunaga et al. [6] reported a woman at 28 weeks of pregnancy with a defect of previous myomectomy scar. The defect was sutured and the pregnancy was continued. Elective caesarean section was carried out at 34 weeks.

Sutton and co-authors [10] reported a 44-year-old woman with previous fundal myomectomy who presented with acute pain abdomen. The diagnosis was established 12 h after admission when an emergency classical caesarean was done to deliver a live foetus. Dim and co-authors [2] reported yet another interesting case where a large fundal rupture of the uterus was diagnosed in a primigravida. She had undergone adenomyomectomy 11 months prior. The rupture was diagnosed 12 h after delivery.

Bernardi et al. [1] studied the outcome of laparoscopic myomectomies and reported a uterine rupture rate of 10 %. In the study by Tian and colleagues [12], the finding of scar defect was higher after laparoscopic myomectomy compared to transabdominal myomectomy where none of the cases had a defect. The authors have therefore recommended limited use of electrocautery during laparoscopic myomectomy. Pistofidis and colleagues [8] analysed the seven cases of uterine ruptures after laparoscopic myomectomies reported to the Board of Endoscopic Gynaecological Surgery over a 13-year period. They observed that haemostasis was achieved by bipolar diathermy alone in nearly 30 % of the cases. 86 % of cases were likely to have been exposed to over diathermy. Two-layered closure of the bed with sutures had been performed in only 14 % of cases. The interval between myomectomy and pregnancy was about 1.4 years. Uterine rupture was mostly seen after 34 weeks and during labour in about 14 % cases.

In a review of 19 cases of rupture of the uterus after laparoscopic myomectomy, Parker and colleagues [7] found that 17 cases had use of cautery during myomectomy. The authors recommended limited use of cautery and layered closure with suture during laparoscopic myomectomy. In the case reported by Kislei and colleagues [4], the woman experienced acute pain in the abdomen and went on to develop foetal distress as early as 23 weeks of pregnancy. She had undergone laparoscopic myomectomy a year earlier.

Thus, a high index of suspicion of ruptured uterus in subsequent pregnancies is needed in a woman who has undergone a myoma removal procedure. It is important to be vigilant for symptoms of pain including shoulder tip pain as a warning symptom. Prompt laparotomy when rupture is suspected would reduce the maternal morbidity and perinatal mortality.

References

1. Bernardi TS, Radosa MP, Weisheit A, Diebolder H, Schneider U, Schleussner E, Runnebaum IB. Laparoscopic myomectomy: a 6-year follow-up single-center cohort analysis of fertility and obstetric outcome measures. Arch Gynecol Obstet. 2014;290(1):87–91. doi:10.1007/s00404-014-3155-2. Epub 2014 Feb 7.
2. Dim CC, Agu PU, Dim NR, Ikeme AC. Adenomyosis and uterine rupture during labour in a primigravida: an unusual obstetric emergency in Nigeria. Trop Doct. 2009;39(4):250–1. doi:10.1258/td.2009.080359.
3. Djaković I, Rudman SS, Kosec V. Uterine rupture following myomectomy in the third trimester. Acta Clin Croat. 2015;54(4):521–4.
4. Kiseli M, Artas H, Armagan F, Dogan Z. Spontaneous rupture of the uterus in mid-trimester pregnancy due to increased uterine pressure with previous laparoscopic myomectomy. Int J Fertil Steril. 2013;7(3):239–42. Epub 2013 Sep 18.
5. Lenihan M, Krawczyk A, Canavan C. Shoulder-tip pain as an indicator of uterine rupture with a functioning epidural. Int J Obstet Anesth. 2012;21(2):200–1. doi:10.1016/j.ijoa.2012.01.004. Epub 2012 Mar 6.
6. Matsunaga J, Daly CB, Bochner CJ, Agnew CL. Repair of uterine dehiscence with the continuation of pregnancy. Obstet Gynecol. 2004;104(5 Pt 2):1211–2.
7. Parker WH, Einarsson J, Istre O, Dubuisson JB. Risk factors for uterine rupture after laparoscopic myomectomy. J Minim Invasive Gynecol. 2010;17(5):551–4. doi:10.1016/j.jmig.2010.04.015. Epub 2010 Jun 29.
8. Pistofidis G, Makrakis E, Balinakos P, Dimitriou E, Bardis N, Anaf V. Report of 7 uterine rupture cases after laparoscopic myomectomy: update of the literature. J Minim Invasive Gynecol. 2012;19(6):762–7. doi:10.1016/j.jmig.2012.07.003.
9. Song SY, Yoo HJ, Kang BH, Ko YB, Lee KH, Lee M. Two pregnancy cases of uterine scar dehiscence after laparoscopic myomectomy. Obstet Gynecol Sci. 2015;58(6):518–21. Published online 2015 Nov 16. doi: 10.5468/ogs.2015.58.6.518.
10. Sutton C, Standen P, Acton J, Griffin C. Spontaneous uterine rupture in a preterm pregnancy following myomectomy. Case Rep Obstet Gynecol. 2016;2016:6195621. doi:10.1155/2016/6195621. Epub 2016 Jan 26.
11. Tauchi M, Hasegawa J, Oba T, Arakaki T, Takita H, Nakamura M, Sekizawa A. A case of uterine rupture diagnosed based on routine focused assessment with sonography for obstetrics. J Med Ultrason (2001). 2016;43(1):129–31. doi:10.1007/s10396-015-0662-0. Epub 2015 Sep 3.
12. Tian YC, Long TF, Dai YM. Pregnancy outcomes following different surgical approaches of myomectomy. Obstet Gynaecol Res. 2015;41(3):350–7. doi:10.1111/jog.12532. Epub 2014 Sep 26.

Rupture Due to Gestational Trophoblastic Disease

7

A woman was admitted with a diagnosis of molar pregnancy in her third pregnancy. She presented in her 4th month of pregnancy due to spotting from the vagina. At admission, she was mildly anaemic. Abdomen revealed a uterine size of 32 weeks with no foetal parts. Sonography confirmed a complete mole. She was planned for elective evacuation after all the preoperative investigations were done. A consultant uneventfully completed the suction evacuation. 2 h after the procedure, she was found to be tachypneic and pale. Her pulse was 120/min, and blood pressure was 90 mm of Hg systolic. She had tachypnea and dyspnea. Abdomen appeared distended. Initially, I thought that she has gone in for adult respiratory distress syndrome due to metastases of the mole, but the abdominal distension was not fitting into the diagnosis. I decided to do a scan, and to my surprise, I found that the uterus which was found to be 12 weeks size showed a possible invasion by the molar tissue on the anterior wall. We took her up for laparotomy as in spite of resuscitation her condition did not stabilize.

There was a 3×4 cm irregular perforated area on the anterior wall through which molar tissue was protruding (Fig. 7.1), and there was brisk bleeding from the partially ruptured myometrium.

We proceeded with hysterectomy. I presume that it was not perforation at the procedure of evacuation, but the invasion of the myometrium by the molar tissue (confirmed so by histopathology) which caused the weakening, and the brisk bleed got precipitated following the handling during the evacuation procedure. She later required chemotherapy due to persistent trophoblastic disease.

The following case once again makes me wonder why a few women are not fated to have their children. She was a case of the recurrent mole. In the first pregnancy, the mole was evacuated uneventfully, and the follow-up was uneventful. In the second conception after 2 years, she was diagnosed with repeat molar pregnancy. The same was evacuated, but she developed the persistent gestational trophoblastic disease and feature suggestive of an invasive mole in the uterus. She underwent chemotherapy. There was complete clearance with undetectable βhCG levels for nearly 2 years. She attempted pregnancy again. This time, she presented at 10 weeks of

© Springer Nature Singapore Pte Ltd. 2017
G. Dorairajan, *Ruptured Uterus*, DOI 10.1007/978-981-10-2852-6_7

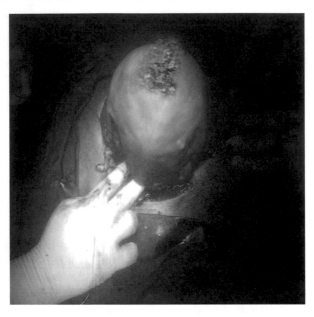

Fig. 7.1 Intraoperative photograph showing molar tissue perforating from the fundus of the uterus

pregnancy in shock with haemoperitoneum. Urgent laparotomy confirmed rupture of the uterus with invasive molar tissue. Hysterectomy was carried out. She underwent multidrug chemotherapy (EMA-CO regimen). It has been now two years, and her βhCG levels have been undetectable for the last 6 months.

Bruner and colleagues [2] reported a woman who presented with rupture due to gestational trophoblastic neoplasia 1 month after the evacuation of molar pregnancy. Their patient had only tachycardia. She was neither very pale nor had low blood pressure. The diagnosis was confirmed on contrast CT scan of the pelvis which confirmed blood around the heterogeneous uterus.

Boufettal and Samouh [1] reported a multigravida admitted in haemorrhagic shock due to rupture of uterus filled with molar pregnancy. Sánchez-Ferrer and colleagues [5] reported another interesting case of complete hydatidiform with twin live foetus. Histopathology and other techniques proved it. Since the twin foetus was alive and morphologically normal and had a normal karyotype, so the pregnancy was opted to be continued after counselling. However, she had rupture of the uterus at 15 weeks of pregnancy requiring a hysterectomy. She later required chemotherapy for the persistent trophoblastic disease. In yet another case reported by Ozdemir et al. [4], the woman presented with features of rupture due to placenta percreta at 21 weeks. She had two previous molar pregnancies for which suction evacuation and curettage had been done. The rupture was managed by suturing with two layers. The abnormal placentation in the index pregnancy could be due to the curettage or may be due to the gestational trophoblastic disease causing weakening of the myometrium.

Kaczmarek and co-authors [3] reported intrapartum rupture and foetal death in a woman who had been earlier treated with chemotherapy for gestational trophoblastic neoplasia with chemotherapy. Though this case has been reported nearly 20 years back, it is worth mentioning for the rarity and for bringing out the need for vigilance in such cases during subsequent pregnancies.

Thus, one has to be vigilant about ruptured uterus in a woman with an ongoing invasive mole as well as a woman who has had a previous gestational trophoblastic disease where the invading molar tissue might have weakened the uterus and can rupture in subsequent pregnancy and labour.

References

1. Boufettal H, Samouh N. Uterine rupture during a hydatidiform mole. Pan Afr Med J. 2014;18:293. doi:10.11604/pamj.2014.18.293.5055. 14. French.
2. Bruner DI, Pritchard AM, Clarke J. Uterine rupture due to the invasive metastatic gestational trophoblastic neoplasm. West J Emerg Med. 2013;14(5):444–7. doi:10.5811/westjem.2013.4.15868.
3. Kaczmarek JC, Kates R, Rau F, Kohorn E, Curry S. Intrapartum uterine rupture in a primiparous patient previously treated for invasive mole. Obstet Gynecol. 1994;83(5 Pt 2):842–4.
4. Ozdemir A, Ertas IE, Gungorduk K, Kaya C, Solmaz U, Yildirim G. Uterine preservation in placenta percreta complicated by unscarred uterine rupture at the second trimester in a patient with repeated molar pregnancies: a case report and brief review of the literature. Clin Exp Obstet Gynecol. 2014;41(5):590–2 ISSN: 0390–6663.
5. Sánchez-Ferrer ML, Hernández-Martínez F, Machado-Linde F, Ferri B, Carbonel P, Nieto-Diaz A. Uterine rupture in twin pregnancy with normal fetus and complete hydatidiform mole. Gynecol Obstet Invest. 2014;77(2):127–33. doi:10.1159/000355566. Epub 2013 Oct 17.

Ruptured Uterus in Gynaecological Situations

8

Perforations after surgical abortions or curettage are complications that most of the gynaecologists would have come across and managed. Fortunately, the perforations following illegal abortions with injuries to internal organs and frank peritonitis are on the decrease with the advent of medical methods of abortion.

As a special mention, I would like to bring out two rare presentations of rupture uterus.

I got a call from the emergency operation theatre by the registrar of surgery. They had opened up the abdomen of a 50-year-old postmenopausal lady admitted with a diagnosis of peritonitis. One litre of pus had been drained. They found a rent in the anterior wall of the uterus. All other organs were normal. The patient was under general anaesthesia in the supine position. There was no way to gather any more information. There was a 2 cm ragged rent in the anterior wall (Fig. 8.1). There was no obvious growth protruding from the rent. I decided to proceed with hysterectomy. When I was clamping to reach the cardinal ligaments, I realized that it is an advanced cancer cervix with induration of the cardinal ligament. Fortunately vesicovaginal plane was free. I could accomplish total hysterectomy and kept my fingers crossed that there should be no reactionary haemorrhage or infection. The cervix had an indurated growth. Fortunately, she had an uneventful recovery. The histopathology confirmed squamous cell carcinoma of the cervix. She received postoperative radiotherapy after complete wound healing. The learning point for all those in the emergency room is to have the cervix evaluated by a clinical examination in every woman with a surgical problem.

A similar case was reported by Shapey et al. [5]. An 84-year-old woman was diagnosed with peritonitis. She was suspected to have diverticulitis of the colon. But at laparotomy, there was perforation of the anterior wall of the uterus which was due to a large leiomyoma of the posterior wall that had undergone hyaline change.

In yet another case of a 46-year-old woman diagnosed with peritonitis, laparotomy revealed a necrosed perforated anterior wall which was confirmed to be due to endometrial carcinoma by histopathology [2].

© Springer Nature Singapore Pte Ltd. 2017
G. Dorairajan, *Ruptured Uterus*, DOI 10.1007/978-981-10-2852-6_8

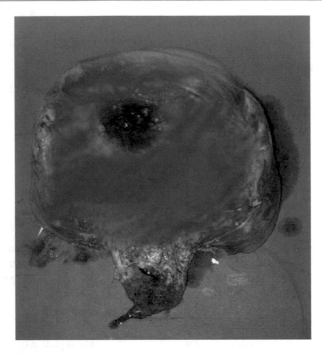

Fig. 8.1 The hysterectomy specimen of the woman with peritonitis showing perforated uterus due to pyometra that occurred due to underlying cancer of the uterine cervix

Weng and colleagues [9] reported a 71-year-old woman with abdominal sepsis. Laparotomy revealed a rupture of the anterior wall of the uterus that was confirmed to be due to infarction of the myometrium. It was probably due to comorbid medical conditions that had caused atherosclerosis of uterine arterioles and ischaemia.

The following case I encountered was a very rare manifestation. A 42-year-old woman presented with severe pain in the lower abdomen. She was a known case of a fibroid uterus. She was asymptomatic. She had been following up. The fibroid was about 8 cm for the last 2 years. It was arising from the anterior wall. During the presentation with acute pain, there was tachycardia. Her blood pressure was normal. She was not anaemic. Abdomen revealed tender lower abdomen with guarding. There was an ill-defined mass in the hypogastrium. We initially thought there is degeneration of the myoma. She was admitted and managed with parenteral analgesics. However, her symptoms and signs did not settle. So the decision for surgery was taken. On opening the abdomen, there was minimal reactionary fluid in the abdomen with flimsy omentum adhesions to the uterus. The leiomyoma had perforated from the anterior wall of the uterus (Fig. 8.2). A total abdominal hysterectomy was carried out. There was no evidence of any malignancy.

Peng et al. [3] reported a nulliparous 39-year-old woman with acute internal bleeding and uterine masses. Laparotomy confirmed a rupture at the posterior cervical-uterine junction. The uterus was extremely enlarged with several leiomyoma and adenomyosis of the posterior wall. There was no history of prior surgeries

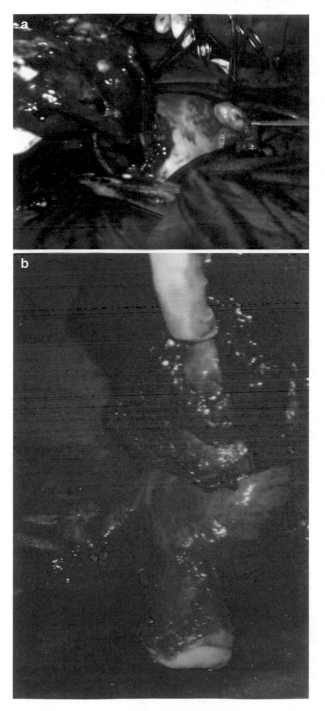

Fig. 8.2 (**a**) Intraoperative photograph showing the perforating leiomyoma. (**b**) The hysterectomy specimen showing the perforated leiomyoma

or curettage. Ramskill and co-authors [4] reported a uterine rupture secondary to a fibroid in a 33-year-old woman in labour. She had no previous surgeries or abortion.

Spontaneous rupture of a degenerated fibroid was reported by Tan and Naidu [8] in a 31-year-old woman after 9 weeks of delivery. She had presented with severe pain abdomen. Imaging confirmed a posterior wall fibroid with a lot of free fluid. Exploratory laparotomy confirmed the rupture and bleeding from it. Myomectomy and suturing were successfully performed.

Bastu et al. [1] reported a 48-year-old nulliparous woman with acute pain abdomen. At laparotomy, she had 2 litres of haemoperitoneum and a large fibroid (smooth muscle tumour of unknown malignant potential) which had undergone cystic degeneration and had ruptured. Takai and colleagues reported a similar case [7].

Shashoua and colleagues have reported rupture of the uterus due to ischaemia three months after uterine artery embolization. The women required a hysterectomy [6].

Thus, rupture uterus could happen outside the setting of pregnancy or labour. It invariably presents with features of acute abdomen though there may not be associated hypovolemia due to haemorrhage.

References

1. Bastu E, Akhan SE, Ozsurmeli M, Galandarov R, Sozen H, Gungor-Ugurlucan F, Iyibozkurt AC. Acute hemorrhage related to spontaneous rupture of a uterine fibroid: a rare case report. Eur J Gynaecol Oncol. 2013;34(3):271–2.
2. Kurashina R, Shimada H, Matsushima T, Doi D, Asakura H, Takeshita T. Spontaneous uterine perforation due to clostridial gas gangrene associated with endometrial carcinoma. Nippon Med Sch. 2010;77(3):166–9.
3. Peng CR, Chen CP, Wang KG, Wang LK, Chen YY, Chen CY. Spontaneous rupture and massive hemoperitoneum from uterine leiomyomas and adenomyosis in a nongravid and unscarred uterus. Taiwan J Obstet Gynecol. 2015;54(2):198–200. doi:10.1016/j.tjog.2014.03.004.
4. Ramskill N, Hameed A, Beebeejaun Y. Spontaneous rupture of uterine leiomyoma during labour. BMJ Case Rep. 2014;2014:pii: bcr2014204364. doi:10.1136/bcr-2014-204364.
5. Shapey IM, Nasser T, Dickens P, Haldar M, Solkar MH. Spontaneously perforated pyometra: an unusual cause of acute abdomen and pneumoperitoneum. Ann R Coll Surg Engl. 2012;94(8):e246–8. doi:10.1308/003588412X13373405387410.
6. Shashoua AR, Stringer NH, Pearlman JB, Behmaram B, Stringer EA. Ischemic uterine rupture and hysterectomy 3 months after uterine artery embolization. J Am Assoc Gynecol Laparosc. 2002;9(2):217–20.
7. Takai H, Tani H, Matsushita H. Rupture of a degenerated uterine fibroid as a cause of acute abdomen: a case report. J Reprod Med. 2013;58(1–2):72–4.
8. Tan YL, Naidu A. Rare postpartum ruptured degenerated fibroid: a case report. J Obstet Gynaecol Res. 2014;40(5):1423–5. doi:10.1111/jog.12334. Epub 2014 Apr 2.
9. Weng LC, Menon T, Hool G. Spontaneous rupture of the non-gravid uterus. BMJ Case Rep. 2013;2013:pii: bcr2013008895. doi:10.1136/bcr-2013-008895.

Management and Complications

9

Management of ruptured uterus depends on the cause, the presentation, the need to preserve the uterus, and the part of the uterus involved in the rupture.

Resuscitation is a very important first aid and must be initiated as soon as rupture is suspected. Effective resuscitation to keep the blood pressure above 90 mm of Hg systolic is a very important step to prevent postoperative complications. Initial resuscitation with crystalloids (maximum up to 1.5 l in 1 h) and blood is necessary. Overuse of crystalloids without blood would result in dilution and consumption coagulopathy, compounding the bleeding. However, resuscitation and preparation for definitive surgical management should be carried out parallel. Delay beyond 1 h from diagnosis is likely to result in the life-threatening sequel and even death. With abnormal foetal heart rate pattern in a woman with a previous caesarean scar in labour, the time delay beyond 15 min to a half hour would result in perinatal mortality. It is important to ensure round-the-clock availability of blood, anaesthetist and operation theatre facility, and skilled obstetricians before planning the delivery of women with higher risk of rupture like women with a previously scarred uterus.

Most of the ruptures associated with previous lower segment caesarean sections have a subacute maternal presentation with the rupture restricted to the lower segment. Most of these are amenable to repair. Repair should always be attempted and is most likely to be successful when the rupture is restricted to the lower segment and is a fresh rupture. In a study period of 10 years, Alemayehu and co-authors [1] observed that 98 % of cases with rupture were successfully repaired by the doctors even though they were nonspecialized doctors. The authors further observed that the maternal mortality increases sevenfold if there is more than 1 h delay in definitive treatment.

One needs to keep in mind the recurrence of rupture in subsequent pregnancies. Eshkoli and co-authors [3] observed a recurrent risk of rupture to be 15 %. Fox et al. [4] studied the outcome of pregnancies with previous ruptures and observed that those who had a dehiscence of scar in the previous pregnancy or labour had a higher risk of repeat dehiscence at 7.5 %. However, they observed that management of these patients with standard protocol by repeat elective caesarean sections would not increase the maternal or perinatal morbidity or mortality.

© Springer Nature Singapore Pte Ltd. 2017
G. Dorairajan, *Ruptured Uterus*, DOI 10.1007/978-981-10-2852-6_9

In situations where there is associated colporrhexis or extension of the rupture to the lateral wall, a hysterectomy might become necessary. In a population-based study spanning over 23 years, Charach and Sheiner [2] recorded 164 ruptures and observed that the woman is likely to have a hysterectomy if she is subjected to relaparotomy, if there is an extension of a tear to cervix or fornix, if there is continued bleeding requiring multiple transfusions, and if she is a multiparous woman.

Ruptures involving the upper segment invariably merit a hysterectomy. Similarly, tears of the lateral wall involving the uterine artery or bleeding into the broad ligament are also likely to require a hysterectomy. Repair can be attempted if the tear is linear, but future pregnancies should be avoided as the risk of subsequent rupture is very high, and so tubal ligation should be performed along with repair after counselling. If the rupture is due to an invasive mole or the margins are ragged, and there is a loss of tissue, hysterectomy becomes necessary.

Caesarean hysterectomy is a skilled procedure. The surgery needs to be very fast. Preoperative urinary catheterization is must to not only rule out bladder rupture but also aid in the diagnosis of urinary tract injuries during the surgery as the chances of urinary tract injuries are high during caesarean hysterectomy, and of course, urine output during the surgery is an important measure of effective maintenance of circulation. In women suspected with a rupture, the abdomen should be preferably opened by vertical midline sub-umbilical incision. After the foetus and placenta are extracted from the abdominal cavity, the uterus should be delivered out and inspected for the site and size of rupture, the condition of the edges, the involvement of the uterine arteries, and the bleeding from the edges, as also for broad ligament bleeding in situations involving the lateral wall and the uterine arteries.

One needs to keep in mind that engorged distended vasculature of pregnancy can result in brisk bleeding and there is a higher chance of retraction of the uterine artery. Though working at the level of the abdominal wall with the enlarged uterus and tissue oedema makes the exposure and the identification of the tissue plane easier. One also needs to regard the fact that ruptures older than 12 h are likely to be associated with oedema of the ruptured edges and are likely to result in cut through making the repair difficult. Rupture following obstructed or neglected labour is likely to be associated with thinned-out friable edges and sometimes infected edges making any attempt at repair futile and frustrating.

The caesarean hysterectomy typically starts with clamping, cutting, and ligating the tubo-ovarian ligaments. The ovaries should be preserved. Tissue oedema and engorged vessels pose a serious threat for making the ligature loose so they should be tightened securely. The next clamp is in the structures of broad ligament including the round ligament. The utero-vesical fold of peritoneum is identified and incised to push the bladder down.

In situations where the utero-vesical fold has been already incised to perform lower segment caesarean section, the first step could be to clamp, cut, and ligate the round ligaments. The urinary bladder is further pushed down. One has to be careful at this step as the lower segment may be thinned out friable or the bladder itself may be oedematous and pulled up especially in cases with lateral wall ruptures following neglected labour. During pregnancy, the venous plexuses supplying the bladder are engorged and prominent and might bleed when pushing the bladder on the sides. Clamps are now applied at the level of the isthmus to the uterine arteries. The uterine arteries have a tendency to retract on cutting so the pedicle should be kept thick and double clamping may be necessary at the proximal stump. This drastically reduces the blood loss. The tubo-ovarian ligament is then clamped, cut, and ligated.

After uterine artery ligation, progressively medial clamps are applied parallel to the uterine cervix on the cardinal ligament and then the vaginal angles. The cervix can be felt as a bulge or with a finger guided within the cavity of the uterus from the tear. Sometimes cervix may be difficult to identify when the uterus gets avulsed or when the rupture has happened in the second stage. If the patient is in shock and poor circulation, subtotal hysterectomy may be sufficient if that serves the purpose of haemostasis as it saves a lot of time.

In a subtotal hysterectomy, after the uterine artery ligation, we need to direct the next clamp, towards the lower segment or the cervix. The same can be cut with a knife and the cervix is sutured anteroposteriorly.

The other technique is "cut and go" where serial clamps are applied and cut from the tubo-ovarian ligament downwards till the uterine arteries to achieve quick arrest of bleeding. The clamps are replaced by ligatures after all the clamps have been applied above downwards. However, this has the disadvantage that not all the laparotomy trays will have so many clamps readily available and too many clamps may create clutter in the operative field and any jumping clamp could make the situation worse and result in a struggle to hold back the pedicles. Once all the pedicles have been ligated, one should double-check for any bleeders. There is a higher risk of injury to the urinary tract during surgery. Blind haemostatic sutures without skeletonizing and identifying the bleeder in the broad ligament or near the vault pose a significant threat to the ureters. Guiding the hand to lift the posterior leaf of broad ligament after identifying the ureter and ensuring it is away from the field can prevent such inadvertent injury to the distal third of the ureter. If there is any doubt about bladder integrity, it can be checked by retrograde filling with methylene blue or opaque sterile fluid or intravenous indigo carmine injection. If the haemostasis is good, closing blood pressure is normal, and there is no feature of consumption coagulopathy, then usually intraperitoneal drain is not necessary.

The complications of rupture of the uterus include shock, acute tubular necrosis of kidney consequent to the shock, consumption coagulopathy, hypoxic brain damage, ischaemic necrosis of the posterior pituitary, and sepsis. Quick exsanguination can cause death. Multiple transfusions can further compound the situation with acute lung injury, pulmonary oedema, and haemolysis. There is a high risk of thromboembolism due to anaemia, prolonged surgery, immobilization, hypercoagulability of pregnancy, and supervening sepsis.

Effective and prompt resuscitation, definitive surgical treatment without delay, broad-spectrum antibiotics, and prompt but prudent use of blood and products will prevent most of these complications. Prolonged catheterization and rest to the bladder may be necessary depending on the cause of rupture and the intraoperative condition of the urinary bladder.

Remote complications include anaemia, chronic pelvic pain, psychological trauma, and the sequel-like Sheehan syndrome. Urinary fistulae can form in a woman who has had neglected labour prior to rupture.

A high index of suspicion, early recognition, prompt resuscitation, prompt surgery without delay, and gentle handling of tissues would reduce the mortality and morbidity. Intensive monitoring in the post operative period, appropriate replacement of fluids, blood and components, and antibiotics is necessary for smooth recovery. Early recognition and appropriate treatment of threatening complications would further reduce the mortality and the long-term morbidity.

References

1. Alemayehu W, Ballard K, Wright J. Primary repair of obstetric uterine rupture can be safely undertaken by non-specialist clinicians in rural Ethiopia: a case series of 386 women. BJOG. 2013;120(4):505–8.
2. Charach R, Sheiner E. Risk factors for peripartum hysterectomy following uterine rupture. J Matern Fetal Neonatal Med. 2013;26(12):1196–200 (ISSN: 1476–4954).
3. Eshkoli T, Weintraub AY, Baron J, Sheiner E. The significance of a uterine rupture in subsequent births. Arch Gynecol Obstet. 2015;292(4):799–803.
4. Fox NS, Gerber RS, Mourad M, Saltzman DH, Klauser CK, Gupta S, Rebarber A. Pregnancy outcomes in patients with prior uterine rupture or dehiscence. Obstet Gynecol. 2014;123(4):785–9.

Printed in the United States
By Bookmasters